Contents

Implementation of the Global Strategy for Health for All by the Year 2000

SECOND EVALUATION

Eighth report on the world health situation

VOLUME 1 GLOBAL REVIEW

WHO Library Cataloguing in Publication Data

Implementation of the global strategy for health for all by the year 2000 : second evaluation : eighth report on the world health situation.

  Contents: v. 1. Global review

  1.Health plan implementation – trends   2.Health policy – trends   3.Health status   4.World health   II.Title:
  Eighth report on the world health situation

  ISBN 92 4 160281 3 (v.1)   (NLM Classification: WA 540.1)

93/9601 – Schüler – 5200

Preface

I am pleased to present to the scientific community and to decision-makers in the health and health-related sectors, the Eighth Report on the World Health Situation, prepared on the basis of the second evaluation of the Global Strategy for Health for All by the Year 2000. It is primarily a synthesis of findings from reports of Member States who carried out their evaluation in 1991 – the second time since the Global Strategy was adopted by the World Health Assembly in 1981 – and consists of a global review and six regional reports.

The period 1985–1990 covered by the report was characterized by dramatic changes in both the political and the economic situations. On the positive side, there was a widespread move towards democratization of political systems and greater participation of people in determining their own future. Human rights, equity and social justice increasingly became basic concerns in the political decision-making process. The expression of individual and ethnic rights, however, led to increased violence and local conflicts and strife in some countries. Economic policy also changed drastically and there was an increasing trend towards recognizing the importance of health as a basic element of development. However, it was the least developed countries which faced difficulties even in maintaining basic minimum services in the social sectors, including health.

And yet, the period witnessed perceptible improvements in health care coverage and health status, though such progress has been un-even, differing in various parts of the world, among population groups within countries and in different age groups. While commitment to the aims of health for all has remained firm and Member States have adopted the primary health care approach as described in the Declaration of Alma-Ata for the development of their health care systems, the implementation of strategies to achieve those aims has in many cases slowed down. This slowing down has resulted not only from economic factors but also from the rigidity of health systems, weak infrastructure, the constraints on achieving real participation by all related sectors and the inadequacy of efforts to promote health and prevent specific health problems.

At the same time, the developing countries have been experiencing an epidemiological transition, with rapid aging of the population together with an increasing incidence of noncommunicable diseases linked to changes in lifestyle. The growing prevalence of cancer, cardiovascular disease, diabetes and other chronic conditions in addition to the long-standing problems of communicable diseases such as cholera, malaria and tuberculosis impose a double burden on health care systems in these countries. There are also worrying trends in mortality from accidents and suicide in young adults, particularly in the developed countries. In addition, there is the pandemic of HIV infection and AIDS, which imposes a particularly heavy burden on developing countries. All these realities must be taken into account in implementing public health action geared to achieving the goal of health for all through primary health care.

The dream of health for all is slowly – perhaps too slowly – becoming a reality. We must evolve and develop new approaches, new mechanisms, new partnerships and new resources that can expedite this process. The problems now being faced may not be susceptible to approaches that have been applied in the past. We cannot continue doing what we have always done. Tomorrow cannot be just more of yesterday. We need flexibility and pragmatism as much as innovation but the stress must invariably be on *action*.

This global review and the six regional reports provide information for defining an *implementation* framework for new public health action for accelerating progress in achieving the goal of health for all. It is only when this is translated into action that we can say it has served its purpose.

DIRECTOR-GENERAL

Executive summary

The report on the implementation of the Global Strategy for Health for All by the Year 2000, second evaluation, and eighth report on the world health situation, consists of a global review and six regional reports. The global review is derived principally from national and regional evaluation reports. Where necessary, information from other sources has been used, especially from WHO programmes and from documents of other international organizations. The information used relates primarily to the period 1985–1990 which is covered by this evaluation. Some developments which occurred after this period may not have been fully reflected therefore, however significant they may be. The evaluation on which this review is based has so far been characterized by the greater preparedness of countries than for the earlier review; they were more involved in the process and more thorough. Countries seem to have felt that this was their own evaluation, rather than just WHO's. This is illustrated by the response rate: 151 countries out of 168 submitted reports, covering 5200 million people (or 96% of the world population).

Chapter 1 (Global trends in socioeconomic development) focuses on the interrelation of political, economic, demographic and social development trends and their implications for health for the period 1985–1990. There has been a noticeable trend among governments and international development agencies towards the recognition of people as the centre of development, and health as a basic component thereof.

The social and political dimensions of development have also received more attention from international development organizations and agencies. The global environment is becoming more favourable to decision-making in health, given the general global trend towards democracy and freedom, initiatives such as universal literacy by the year 2000, and the integration of women in the mainstream of development policies. In health development there is a general trend towards more involvement of individuals, communities, professional groups and development agencies. Adult literacy rate and per capita gross national products (GNP) have increased globally, including those in the developing countries and the least developed among them (LDCs), although not significantly for the latter.

The global economic environment, however, was unable to support sustainable national socioeconomic development owing to the slowing down of the pace of economic growth in the 1980s, increasing balance of payments problems in many countries, growing disparities in the production performances in different parts of the world, and emerging new trade and foreign debt policies and practices. As far as health care financing is concerned, a number of developing countries have retained traditional systems established during former colonial times. The national socioeconomic environment has thus not generally been conducive to the development of health systems based on primary health care, particularly where civil strife and sociopolitical instability have prevailed.

Changes in priorities were also noted as a result of the global recession, natural or man-made disasters and other emerging or new problems such as cholera and AIDS. The developing countries, particularly the LDCs, have been looking for ways to make judicious use of the available national and international aid resources to implement their policies and strategies.

Chapter 2 (Development of health systems) focuses on the progress made in countries in achieving the objective of health for all, namely to reduce the gaps between the "haves" and the "have nots". Overall there has been strong political commitment to achieving health-for-all goals, and most countries have endorsed at the highest level the health-for-all policies and strategies. Mechanisms to involve people are reported to be fully functioning or are being further developed in most countries, and policy decisions have thus been taken in many countries, enabling them to mobilize at least central government resources for health. However, in implementing the strategy, the fundamental health-for-all policies and the principles applicable to health systems based on primary health care (PHC) have not always been put into practice in appropriate ways by the countries when attempting to facilitate universal access to essential health care with all eight essential elements of PHC on a continuing basis. The factors that slowed progress in implementing the strategy were: (1) the slow pace with which existing disease-control programmes have been reoriented towards people's needs; (2) problems in bringing together relevant programme activities to provide health care on a continuing basis through the general health infrastructure; (3) difficulties in involving all those concerned (individuals, families, communities and local nongovernmental organizations as well as health personnel) in health care delivery; and (4) weak management of health care delivery, especially at the operational level. The inadequate and uneven distribution of health personnel of different categories has frequently hindered the delivery of an appropriate mix of health care activities. The provision of effective health care directed to specific vulnerable groups and to solving priority problems has been inhibited not only by lack of coordination and integration, but also possibly by lack of managerial expertise and creativity, including insufficient leadership from the ministry of health.

Key factors which have consistently been identified in the successful development of health systems were: government, political, social and financial commitment; strong management capabilities for implementation; well-oriented, trained and committed health personnel; decentralization; community involvement; sustained financing; and widespread availability of affordable technology.

Chapter 3 (Health care) reviews progress and constraints in health care coverage, and analyses general trends in coverage by PHC (such as availability and accessibility) and quality of care. The indicator referring to PHC coverage comprises four selected elements of PHC, each of which may cover several subelements (e.g., attendance by trained personnel for women in pregnancy and childbirth, and caring for children up to at least one year of age). Information on the percentage of the population covered by *all* elements of PHC is not available, and the trends in the provision of comprehensive PHC coverage cannot thus be adequately measured. However, globally, significant increases can be seen in the percentage of the population covered by many of the elements and subelements of PHC since the first evaluation in 1985, such as: immunization against the six target diseases of the Expanded Programme on Immunization (EPI); trained personnel at childbirth; local health services; water supply; and excreta disposal facilities. Gaps between the developing and developed countries have been significantly reduced, although improvements in the LDCs have been less satisfactory.

Chapter 4 (Health resources) considers financial resources, human resources and health technology. According to the available data there has been a slight increase in the percentage of GNP spent by central governments for health in all developing countries and most geographical regions. The per capita central government expenditure, however, shows a general fall in real spending in many developing countries. It should be noted that data on central government expenditure on health is difficult to compare among country groupings. There is also evidence that nongovernmental spending on health is becoming increasingly significant. While the percentage of national health expenditure devoted to local health services has been increasing in developed countries, it has been stagnant in the developing countries and has decreased in the LDCs.

From the available data on human resources for health, it appears that the major problem continued to be the maldistribution of health personnel. Many countries are reviewing the relevance of current medical education and assessing different factors which may influence professional behaviour (e.g., environment, remuneration). The administrators of many health programmes, however, continue to train health workers specifically to implement their programme activities and to achieve their particular programme targets. It is also becoming increasingly evident that though there has been expansion of health infrastructure and an improvement in the quality of health personnel, they have not automatically led to any increase in provision of health care because of logistic problems and conditions of employment.

Health technology used in primary health care is still inadequately assessed in most countries. Some countries have reported the establishment of national research priorities related to major diseases or to organizational issues such as human resources and finance. There is, however, no evidence to show that priority has been given to the choice of technology and methods appropriate for effective provision of essential care on a continuing basis through in-tegration of preventive and promotive care with curative and rehabilitative services. This would have operational, financial and ethical implications as well as posing challenges for health professionals, training institutions and health managers.

Chapter 5 (Patterns and trends in health status) reviews developments concerning specific aspects of health status (mortality, morbidity and disability) and of major determinants of health (smoking, alcohol abuse, etc.) and their implications for the achievement of health for all. The epidemiological transition has continued in developing countries, with cardiovascular disease and cancer progressively replacing infectious and parasitic diseases. Tropical diseases seem to have gone on a rampage, with cholera spreading to the Americas for the first time this century, yellow fever and dengue epidemics affecting even greater numbers, the malaria situation deteriorating, schistosomiasis establishing itself in new areas, and leishmaniasis and nonvenereal endemic syphilis increasing. The AIDS pandemic is spreading globally, as also are genital herpes and sexually transmitted chlamydial disease. Pulmonary tuberculosis is on the increase, partly stimulated by combined infection with human immunodeficiency virus (HIV). Pneumonia and hepatitis B remain serious threats. In the developing world, the number of cancer cases has for the first time overtaken that in the developed countries. Lung cancer has overtaken breast cancer as the leading cancer in females in some developed countries owing to the spread of the smoking epidemic among women. Diabetes is increasing everywhere, blindness (especially cataract) is more common, alcohol-related diseases are more frequent, as are mental problems and suicide (particularly in the developed countries). Some diseases of childhood preventable by vaccination – measles, acute paralytic poliomyelitis, pertussis, and neonatal tetanus – are decreasing owing to a rapid increase in coverage by immunization programmes. Cardiovascular diseases in developed countries (except eastern Europe) are on the wane owing to the spread of health education, and lung cancer has begun to decline in males in some developed countries since more men began to give up smoking.

In spite of the increase in many diseases and health problems, the overall death rate and the infant and child mortality rates have continued to decrease globally. This overall progress largely reflects the major gains made against the diseases of early childhood preventable by vaccination and the fact that death from some of the major chronic diseases now occurs later in life.

Chapter 6 (Health and environment) covers environmental health policies and programmes, assessment and monitoring of environmental health hazards and risks, and environmental resources management. Safe water and basic sanitation have been recognized for centuries as major determinants of health. However, only in 1980 was the first major global initiative taken (the International Drinking Water Supply and Sanitation Decade) to mobilize international support and resources so as to provide support to countries in achieving universal access to safe water and basic sanitation. There has also been increasing recognition that the maintenance of life on this planet depends on a delicate balance of forces, which is now threatened by the growth of the human population and its increasing exploitation of limited natural resources leading to pollution of air, soil and water. Concern about deforestation, desertification, depletion of the ozone layer, and climatic change has come to include the health implications of environmental problems of a global nature.

In 1990, the main environmental hazards causing concern remained: urban air pollution (gases, lead, etc.), indoor air pollution, inappropriate use of agrochemicals, contamination of fresh water and drinking-water supplies, hazardous wastes and ionizing radiation. Government awareness of the effects of environmental degradation on health and development has been increasing. The concern of individuals and

groups in many countries is being more clearly expressed, but the health sector has on the whole not been an active party in the process of preventing serious degradation in health status, so as to ensure sustainable development, particularly of human resources.

Chapter 7 (Assessment of achievements) is a synthesis of the previous six chapters, and assesses progress and adequacy in the implementation of the strategies, the effectiveness of health care coverage and results in terms of improved health. It concludes that improvements have been made in health status in terms of life expectancy at birth and infant mortality rates, and in coverage levels by various elements of primary health care. Such improvements seem to be more rapid in the developing countries than in the least developed ones; the disparities in health status between the developed and developing countries have been reduced but the gap between the least developed and other developing countries seems to have increased. There is also some evidence that disparities in health status have increased within countries between certain population groups. In recent years there has not only been a socioeconomic transition but a continuing epidemiological transition towards a predominance of noncommunicable diseases, such as cancer, cardiovascular disease and diabetes, resulting from changes in life-style and the environment and the rapid aging of populations. In addition there has been a resurgence of old scourges, such as tuberculosis and malaria, and the recent emergence of AIDS. Coverage by various elements of primary health care has been unbalanced and distorted; although programmes have achieved their targets, their impact in terms of health status may not be significant. There is also little evidence that international and bilateral funding agencies have significantly shifted their aid priorities towards the low-income and least developed countries.

With the high-level commitment and endorsement of the strategy and the establishment of mechanisms for involving people in efforts to improve health and care, a basis now exists for accelerating implementation. There is also evidence that the health sector has been able to mobilize at least central government resources, in spite of unfavourable economic constraints domestically and internationally. However, it is not yet clear whether resources have actually been equitably distributed and whether available resources have even been significantly shifted to support local health services. Major problems have been insufficient cooperation between programmes within the health sector and inadequate coordination with other sectors. Many countries have been developing innovative ways of financing health care, reviewing their medical education and training programmes for health personnel, and revising disease control programmes to support health protection and promotion.

Chapter 8 (Outlook for the future) draws on the analysis of the preceding chapters, identifies important trends taking place in health and postulates how the trends may develop. It makes a quantitative and qualitative assessment of the future, identifies important strategy issues and updates the challenges posed in the last report on health-for-all monitoring. These five challenges can be enumerated as follows.

The *first* is that renewed accountability by governments to their least favoured populations is called for. They should reconfirm their commitment to equity, especially as regards those populations who have the least access to health care, such as the rural and urban poor, the unemployed, women, children and the elderly. The problems affecting these population groups will also need increased attention.

The *second* stems from the first: redefinition of the roles of governments in health care and reorientation of health systems, taking into account the continuing limits in terms of public resources and management capacity. Health promotion, disease prevention, quality control of care, decentralization and expansion of the private and nongovernmental health care sectors and community roles must all be addressed, as well as the future development of human resources for health to support this orientation.

The *third* is finding enhanced methods of health financing, which will tackle the problems of inequity and inefficiency as well as ethical and human rights aspects, whilst containing and recovering costs, and controlling overall levels of health expenditure. This economic challenge becomes more pressing as the expanding role of the private sector is recognized, and as new blends of government and nongovernmental interaction in the financing and provision of health care develop.

The *fourth* relates to the changing managerial responsibilities in health from political and technical advocacy for health measures to enhanced implementation both within the health sector and among sectors. The role of the health sector in overall social development becomes one of greater support to other sectors, such as education, food and nutrition, and the environment. Communities need to be empowered to assume more responsibility. Public health administration must become more efficient. Management must be strengthened more through appropriate procedures and supervised practice, and less through training, as well as through health information systems more comprehensive in scope.

The *fifth* and final challenge calls for more international cooperation in health. In particular, WHO's collaboration at country level must be enhanced in technical and administrative terms. New styles of collaboration are needed which place technically sound development activities under the management of national staff at different levels. The mobilization of resources for least developed countries must continue and increase. Only through improved technical collaboration with countries can WHO remain the directing and coordinating authority in international health. The function and structure of WHO should be redefined to ensure the rapid and realistic implementation of public health action and sustainable development.

The conclusion relates these trends, issues and challenges to the need for a new framework for sustainable health development directed towards:

- mobilizing resources for high-priority population groups and health needs;
- ensuring equity in health through more effective and intersectoral health promotion and protection;
- pursuing equality in access to primary health care through higher quality and increasingly integrated services not only within the confines of the health services *per se*, but within the entire spectrum of social services.

Introduction

Facing the urgent need to improve the health situation, which was alarming, the Health Assembly decided in 1977 that the main social target of governments and WHO in the coming decades should be "the attainment by all citizens of the world by the year 2000 of a level of health that will permit them to lead a socially and economically productive life", otherwise known as "Health for all by the year 2000" (resolution WHA30.43). Subsequently, the Declaration made at the International Conference on Primary Health Care held in Alma-Ata in 1978 endorsed the goal of health for all by the year 2000 and clearly stated that primary health care is the key to attaining it. All Member States were then invited individually to formulate their own national policies, strategies and plans of action and collectively to formulate regional and global strategies to this end.

In 1981, the Global Strategy (including a short list of indicators for global monitoring and evaluation) was adopted by the World Health Assembly (resolution WHA34.36), and by the United Nations General Assembly (resolution 36/43). In 1982, the Health Assembly approved the plan of action for implementing the Global Strategy (resolution WHA35.23). The plan laid down a timetable for monitoring and evaluation of the Strategy: (1) progress in implementing regional strategies and the Global Strategy was to be monitored every two years by the regional committees and the Executive Board; and (2) effectiveness of the regional strategies and Global Strategy should be evaluated by these same bodies every six years.

The plan of action called on the Director-General to provide support to countries in developing their capacities for monitoring and evaluation and to ensure the collection and analysis of information from countries on the indicators adopted for monitoring and evaluating the Strategy. A common framework was then prepared by WHO for use by countries. The latter meanwhile began setting up suitable monitoring and evaluation processes on this basis.

The first monitoring of progress in implementing the Strategy was carried out in 1983 and the first evaluation of the Strategy in 1985. The *Seventh report on the world health situation*, based on this first evaluation and comprising six regional reports and a global review, was approved by the World Health Assembly in 1986 (resolution WHA39.7). On this occasion, the plan of action was also modified: progress was to be monitored every three years, instead of every two, to allow more time for strengthening the national monitoring and evaluation processes and the related information support systems.

The second monitoring of progress in implementing the Strategy was carried out in 1988 and the global report thereon was adopted by the World Health Assembly in 1989 (resolution WHA42.2). In the same year, the conference "From Alma-Ata to the year 2000 – a midpoint perspective" was held in Riga where experts from WHO and other organizations reviewed progress towards health for all.

The current evaluation

This second evaluation of the implementation of health-for-all strategy covers the period 1985–1990.

There are three main differences between this second evaluation and the first: (1) reformulated global indicators were used; (2) countries were far more closely involved in the process; and, as a result (3) not only was the response-rate better, but the quality of response also improved. In particular, a number of countries provided information on resources, including details about health manpower.

Preparatory activities for the second evaluation began in early 1989. The Executive Board reviewed in 1990 the methodology used by Member States in carrying out the monitoring and evaluation of their strategies and reformulated global indicators to reflect countries' situation (resolution EB85.R5) (see the Annex to this report). A common framework for the second evaluation (CFE/2) was drafted and, on the basis of previous versions and the proposed revised indicators, finalized after testing. Member States used this common framework as a working tool to carry out the evaluation of implementation of their national strategies between the end of September 1990 and the end of January 1991. In accordance with resolution WHA39.7 countries reported on their findings so that the six regional reports/syntheses could be submitted to the regional committees in September–October 1991.

This second evaluation has been characterized by the greater preparedness of countries, which were more involved in the process and more thorough. Countries seem to have felt that this was their own evaluation, rather than just WHO's. Table 1 shows the response rates by countries for the previous monitoring and evaluation exercises, and for the current evaluation, in which 151 countries out of 168 submitted reports, covering 5200 million (or 96% of the population).

The process was improved in the following respects:

- preparatory activities were usually longer, and previous experience was put to good use;
- groups were generally created within the ministry of health, including a variety of personnel from several programmes, as compared with the previous evaluation, where the work was sometimes carried out by consultants;
- the background material used (including material from the previous monitoring) was prepared especially for the evalua-

Table 1

Monitoring and evaluation of the implementation of the strategy for health for all by the year 2000 by WHO member states, 1983–1991

	First monitoring 1983	First evaluation 1985	Second monitoring 1988	Second evaluation 1991
Member States				
Number	160	166	166	168
Reports received	121	147	143	151
Response rate (%)	75.6	88.6	86.1	89.9
Non Member States				
Reports received	1	15	17	9

tion, which moreover in some countries was often based on revised and improved information systems, so that more accurate data were used;

– in a number of countries, joint WHO/ government coordination mechanisms were involved in preparing and/or reviewing the report;

– in some cases, experience from the periphery was specifically sought in an attempt to answer questions on primary health care;

– the reports were carefully summarized by high-level officials before despatch.

Structure and content of the global review

The report on implementation of the Global Strategy for Health for All by the Year 2000, second evaluation, and eighth report on the world health situation, consist of a global review and six regional reports. This global review was prepared on the basis of national and regional evaluation reports, WHO programme information, relevant publications and documents from international agencies and special contributions where necessary. Since the report on the second evaluation had to be submitted to WHO before 31 March 1991, the designations used in this publication are mainly those which applied at that time. Also, due to political developments that took place in the late 1980s and early 1990s, a number of countries were unable to provide WHO with a report on their evaluation.

At the end of 1990, data on global indicators reported in 1983, 1985 and 1988, were sent to regional offices and countries together with estimates for the period covered and for 1991 and 2000 for some of them, for their review and use. Information returned by countries in their reports was synthesized, together with information from WHO technical programmes, and numerical data were validated and checked for consistency. By the end of October 1991, this process had been completed for the 115 reports received according to schedule. Data from 36 reports which were received later were analysed and the global review updated for submission to the World Health Assembly in May 1992. For analytical purposes, countries were classified as developing countries, least developed countries, eastern Europe and developed market economies. The designations of country groups in the text and tables are intended solely for statistical or analytical convenience and do not necessarily express a judgement about the stage reached by a particular country in the development process.

The global review consists of the eight chapters, as follows:

Chapter 1 (Global trends in socioeconomic development) focuses on the interrelationships between political, economic, demographic and social development and their implications for health for the period 1985–1990.

Chapter 2 (Development of health systems) summarizes significant changes, trends and constraints in the development of national health policies and strategies in relation to the Alma-Ata framework, and reviews the organization and development of health systems, managerial processes and mechanisms, community involvement, supporting legislation, intercountry cooperation, and cooperation with WHO and other agencies.

Chapter 3 (Health care) reviews progress and constraints in health care coverage, and analyses general trends in coverage by primary health care (such as availability and accessibility) and quality of care.

Chapter 4 (Health resources) reviews policies and action taken to address various issues concerning the utilization, mobilization and development of resources.

Chapter 5 (Patterns and trends in health status) reviews developments concerning specific aspects of health status (mortality, morbidity and disability) and of major determinants of health (smoking, alcohol abuse, etc.) and their implications for achievement of health for all.

Chapter 6 covers environmental health policies and programmes, assessment and monitoring of environmental health hazards and risks and environmental resources management.

Chapter 7, which is a synthesis of the previous chapters, assesses achievements in terms of progress, adequacy, effectiveness and impact of the Strategy.

Chapter 8 draws from the preceding chapters the major lessons from this evaluation and identifies future trends (generally to the year 2000), the major issues which these trends imply, and the resulting challenges to be addressed in the continuing efforts to achieve national and global health-for-all goals and targets.

How evaluation results can be used

This global review of the world health situation and of the way the Strategy is being implemented by countries may be useful for all those involved in the evaluation, both directly and indirectly, and for those who have an interest in and concern for health.

WHO Member States can use it for a twofold comparison: (1) they can view their present situation in relation to the previous evaluation in order to assess their progress and identify problems, constraints and areas for special attention; and (2) they can observe their own situation in relation to that of other countries within and outside their own Region, and draw on the experience of others. This will enable them to arrive at new solutions to their own problems.

Countries generally reported in more detail about collaborative activities with WHO than with other organizations and agencies concerned with health (e.g., UNDP, UNICEF, UNFPA, various nongovernmental organizations). It is increasingly recognized that for human development, of which health is a basic component, close collaboration amongst international technical and funding agencies is essential. The findings from this evaluation will contribute to an assessment of the health implications of these development activities and of health as a condition for human development.

Apart from forming the basis for the eighth report on the world health situation, this second evaluation will help WHO at all levels to reassess its role in implementing the Strategy (its achievements, adequacy and impact), to focus on specific issues and challenges, and to accelerate its programme activities accordingly. It will also assist in elaborating a framework for new public health action – a paradigm for health – through an analysis and understanding of the health paradigm shift that has resulted from changes in society since the Declaration of Alma-Ata in 1978.

CHAPTER 1

Global trends in socio-economic development[1]

Political trends

As the 1990s began, politically and economically a new world order was gradually emerging. Pessimism surrounding the slow pace of progress in achieving the goals and objectives of the International Development Strategy for the Third United Nations Development Decade (1981–1990) was turning to mild optimism. It was the start of a transition from a relatively simple order in which the majority of nations were more or less dependent on each other to a situation – more complex and less predictable – in which some of the nations or groups within them began taking a leading role. There was an increasing recognition that the security of nations depended as much on economic well-being, social justice, individual rights, and ecological stability as on military prowess.

The cold war that had dominated international affairs for four decades was giving way to a widespread discussion of democracy and development. The trend was towards adopting more democratic forms of government, dismantling rigid central planning systems, and adopting a more market-based and participatory approach. The connection between accountability, the rule of law, openness in decision-making, democratic practice in general, and opportunities for economic efficiency was becoming increasingly apparent (*1,2*).

Namibia became independent and established a multiparty democracy in 1990. With the changes towards racial equity in South Africa, the door was being opened for stability, peace and authentic development in that region. Western countries and the central and eastern European countries were eager to cooperate in achieving international security. The Indian subcontinent on the other hand was more preoccupied than ever with domestic problems (*3*). The east Asia and Pacific area was benefiting from a period of relative stability, with its northern part being free of major wars for the first time in decades. The current political goals in most countries were expressed in terms of respect for individual rights and cultures and sustainable economic growth, and seemed to be contributing to the relative harmony between countries.

The initiatives taken during the last few years to create politico-economic subentities such as the Gulf Cooperation Council, the Union of the Arab Maghreb and the Arab Cooperative Council, either enlarged or followed by the institution of other groups, are examples of the general move towards peace and stability. In Europe, the threat of war was being replaced by the threat of an uncertain future, and the challenge of difficult choices. Hostilities between some ethnic and religious groups erupted in some of the countries where they were previ-

---

1. The information used relates primarily to the period 1985–1990 which is covered by this evaluation. Some developments which occurred after this period may not have been fully reflected therefore, however significant they may be.

ously under control, and continued in several others. New relationships were forming between the European Community and its neighbours in central and eastern Europe, and the desire for effective collaboration to support the economic liberalization was also being fulfilled.

The countries of the South suffered from the effect of a general erosion of the political and economic effectiveness of state and government and those in power were overwhelmed by the combination of internal and external pressures, these often being in competition with one another (4). The South's plea for justice, equity and democracy in the global society was being increasingly understood, and the ending of the cold war presented an opportunity to the Western leaders to complete the process of democratization in Europe, which was a feature of the era following the Second World War, and to concentrate more single-mindedly on developments in the rest of the world (2).

In general the Third World, with a population in 1990 of about 3500 million (about two-thirds of the world population), was also experiencing pressures from emerging popular forces and from leaders seeking policies to speed up development. There was a realization that development needed participation, openness and the stability of the rule of law.

The 1990s seemed to have started with a general desire on the part of people everywhere to participate in and contribute to development, and a willingness to share responsibility as they pursued democratic values and fundamental rights; health could be no exception and the process has already started. With rapid developments in science and technology in health, and with the availability of facilities to communicate information on their benefits and drawbacks, people in the nineties, be they in the South or the North, in developing or developed countries, are demanding better health, longer life expectancy, and the right to choose and decide on a health care environment they desire; they seem to be ready to bear responsibility for

their own health and for contributing more from their own resources.

These changes should have implications for discussions and decisions about health care financing (who must pay, for what, and how much), health technology and research strategy, trade in such commodities as illicit drugs and tobacco, environmental sustainability, etc. The world is preparing to face these challenges individually and collectively; clearly, decision-making in health has to become more open, the condition for real community involvement in health.

Economic trends

World output

The gross world product has risen at an average rate of 3.9% a year during the past three decades when measured at constant 1980 prices and exchange rates. This long-term rise in the capacity of the world economy to supply increasingly diverse kinds of goods and services led to widespread improvements in material standards of living for most of the world's population (5). International trade expanded even faster (at 6% per annum) and significant structural transformations of the world economy occurred, such as an enhancement of the role of market forces in the allocation of resources, the opening up of national economies to international trade, and the implementation of monetary and fiscal policies designed to correct large macro-economic imbalances.

However, during the 1980s, the average pace of economic growth slowed significantly. Increasing balance of payments problems in many countries, and growing disparities in the production performance of different areas of the world, became evident. During the period 1985–1990, gross domestic product grew at about 3.3% per annum for the world as a whole and GDP per capita at about 1.6%; there were, however, perceptible differences in GDP growth rates among geographical regions, with south and east Asia growing at an annual rate of 6.6% compared with western Asia at 0.3%, North Africa at 2.7%, sub-Saharan Africa at 2.3%, and Latin America and the Caribbean at 1.4%. Overall, the gap in per capita GNP between the developed market economies and the developing countries has increased during the period 1985–1990 and, among the latter, between the least developed and other developing countries (see Fig. 1.1, Annex table: global indicator 12).

In spite of globalization and growing interdependence, economic activity in 1990 slowed down in all parts of the world. Unexpected political developments in central and eastern Europe in 1989 and 1990, the crisis in the Middle East, sometimes known in the media as the "Gulf crisis", and recession in several developed market economies generated severe economic shocks and seemed to alter many of the promises for future development. The meagre 1% growth worldwide in 1990 even fell behind world population growth and it was feared that the world economy might not grow at all, resulting in a decline in per capita output in 1991. With a possible rebound in the global output by a modest 2% expected in 1992, the decline in world output per person recorded in 1990 and 1991 would probably be arrested.

In all major country groups, output in 1990 increased more slowly than before or declined in absolute terms. Among major economies, the slowdown was most pronounced in Canada, the United Kingdom and the United States; the Federal Republic of Germany and Japan, however, grew faster than in 1989. Eastern Europe and the USSR have reported the worst drop in economic activity; the economies of eastern Europe as a whole contracted by 11%. In the developing countries, the growth rate was around 3% compared with 3.4% in 1989 and 5% in 1988. Oil-importing developing countries had a major deficit as well (6). In Latin America, output contracted, owing in part to stabilization policies and in part to the slowdown in North America.

In Africa, the growth rate improved but barely enough to keep per capita output from falling; sub-Saharan Africa (excluding Nigeria) had an increase in output of around 2%, but still less than the population growth, and therefore the economic situation worsened.

The crisis in the Middle East affected the region itself profoundly, but in general, oil output expanded rapidly in the countries less directly affected, and the regional aggregate GDP remained unchanged in 1990. In south and southeast Asia, the pace of growth remained higher in 1990, varying between 2.5% and nearly 10%. Although it was affected by the crisis, and despite a fall in growth of exports, it remained the fastest growing region. In countries other than those with developed market economies and where per capita income declined, the population rose from around 700 million in 1989 to 1000 million in 1990, nearly one-fifth of the world's population (6).

Global indicator 12
The per capita gross national product

Fig. 1.1
Average per capita gross national products of countries in various stages of development (global indicator 12), 1985 and 1991

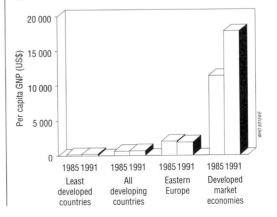

13

An economic performance falling short of apparent potential and resulting in stagnation might be due to shocks beyond the control of individual governments. The necessary adjustments might be costly and time-consuming even in the best of circumstances. As stated in the World Economic Survey (1991), not only were the policies and the theories behind them very much in dispute but the prevailing notions about "sound" policies were being questioned. If economic malaise was widespread, it might be that international economic cooperation had been inadequate. The crisis in the Middle East erupted at a time when the world economy was already showing signs of weakening, so its direct impact on the growth of the world economy is difficult to separate from other influences. The indirect impact of the crisis was probably more important, in so far as it contributed to increased uncertainty about the future and weakened consumer and business confidence (6).

International trade

There was a sharp increase in world trade during 1985–1990, and 1990 was the sixth year in which the increase in world trade exceeded the growth of world output; trade had again become one of the more dynamic elements in the world economy (Table 1.1) (6). However, the rate of growth in 1990 was lower than in 1989, due primarily to much weaker import demand in North America, and to a lesser extent in Japan and the European Economic Community. The volume of imports by countries of central and eastern Europe fell sharply largely due to collapse of trade among members of their Council for Mutual Economic Assistance. Import demand in developing countries remained strong, with growth accelerating in Latin America and in certain countries of south-east Asia and Africa. The sharp fall in primary commodity prices (other than fuels) relative to those of manufactured goods may have caused the slowdown in world economic activity in 1990 and hit mainly the developing countries which are major exporters of primary commodities. World food prices increased slightly, but there were severe declines for coffee, soya beans and wheat; food export prices for developing countries fell by about 6%. Although the prices of agricultural raw materials, led by tropical timber and softwood, increased, as did those for mineral ores, broadly based declines in primary commodity prices were to be expected in 1991 because of the continued slowdown in global economic activity (7).

Both subtle and not-so-subtle policy changes in the international trade environment were noticeable in 1990, and "few of these de-

Table 1.1
Growth rates (%) in GPD, trade volumes, and GDP per capita, 1985–1990

Country groupings	GDP	Trade		GDP per capita
		Export	Import	
World	3.3	6.0	6.2	1.6
Developed market economies	3.0	5.3	6.8	2.5
Central and eastern Europe	2.7	0.4	0.5	1.9
China	8.0	10.3	4.5	6.6
Developing countries	3.4	8.4	6.7	1.0
of which, least developed	3.5	1.0	0.3	0.7

Source: United Nations (1990) and references (5) and (7).

velopments bode well for the future of the liberal and multilateral trading systems" (6). Protectionist tendencies were strenghened and unilateral action began replacing multilateral approaches to resolve trade problems. Through bilateral and regional trade arrangements, the world trading system was being divided into blocks, and trade flows were being diverted towards countries providing more favourable terms. While the deceleration over two or three years in the growth of world trade, mentioned above, need not cause undue concern in the longer term, the delay in concluding the Uruguay Round of multilateral trade negotiations became a cause of anxiety.

International financial resource flows

The most striking observation about the transfer of resources is that, since the early 1980s, most developing countries have been net providers of financial resources to the rest of the world, rather than recipients (6,7). While the current recovery in total resource flows – above US$ 100 billion in 1988 and 1989 – is remarkable for the rising exports of goods and services from developing countries, there has been a marked fall in non-OECD aid and a rise in arrears as a form of finance.[1] Though net official development finance (ODF), including official development assistance (ODA), as well as multilateral and certain bilateral flows increased, in real terms, to US$ 68 billion in 1989, this was largely due to a marked increase in loans at *less concessional* rates loans from bilateral official

sources, particularly the Japanese Export Import bank. Bilateral ODA from Development Assistance Committee donors also increased to US$ 34 billion in 1989 (about 5% in real terms) and total ODA receipts by developing countries remained unchanged in 1989 at US$ 52 billion. However, from the available data it seems that low-income countries were not the primary beneficiaries of aid from international, multilateral and bilateral development agencies (2). In 1990, the developing world as a whole transferred US$ 39 billion abroad (Table 1.2) (6). A surge in the tempo of development will be virtually impossible if the flow of external resources continues to be from the poorer to the richer countries rather than vice versa. Major changes have also been occurring at a time when the ascendancy of finance over industry, together with the globalization of finance, have become the underlying source of instability and unpredictability in the world economy.

International financial institutions are no longer contributing significant net resources to developing countries, and long-term interest rates have been and might continue to be higher than the rates of growth of outputs and exports. As long as the rate of interest is higher than the growth rate of the resources out of which the debt has to be serviced, debt problems, which hit the developing countries much more seriously, will be inevitable. Given that official development assistance might not increase faster than the gross domestic product of the donor countries, where growth has already been slowing down, and that a part of this assistance might be diverted towards eastern Europe as has already happened in the case of food aid, the prospects for development finance for the poorer countries are not bright (6).

Foreign debt of developing countries

The situation of the developing countries as regards debt was not very different in 1990 from what it was in 1980. The aggregate external debt

---

1. *Net resource transfer* includes the net effect of all financial flows in and out of a country including central bank purchase or sale of foreign exchange reserves and all interest and profit flows. *Total net resource flows* to developing countries include official development finance through official development disbursements, total export credits by the Development Assistance Committee and other countries, and private flows covering direct investments by OECD countries, international bank lending, total bond lending, other private sources, and grants by nongovernmental organizations.

Table 1.2

Net transfer of financial resources of groups of developing countries and debt indicators, 1980 and 1985–1990

	1980	1985	1986	1987	1988	1989	1990[a]
Net transfer of resources (billions of dollars)							
All developing countries,	−59.8	−15.3	11.2	−34.1	−24.4	−33.7	−39.0
of which, 15 heavily indebeted countries	8.7	−40.6	−22.1	−28.4	−31.0	−36.2	−30.0
Ratio of external dept to GNP (%)							
All capital importing developing countries	26.4	40.2	42.6	44.0	38.8	35.2	37.3
of which, 15 heavily indebted countries	32.1	57.6	60.8	65.5	55.8	48.9	51.7
Ratio of external debt to exports (%)							
All capital importing developing countries	119.5	176.8	195.2	183.1	154.5	140.3	138.4
of which, 15 heavily indebted countries	168.5	288.7	342.9	334.6	287.3	262.6	248.4
Ratio of debt-service to exports (%)							
All capital importing developing countries	18.6	23.0	23.4	21.9	19.2	15.9	15.8
of which, 15 heavily indebted countries	31.3	37.0	40.8	34.8	36.5	29.1	26.7

[a] Preliminary estimate.
Source: United Nations (1991) and reference (*6*).

rose in 1990 to a new peak of US$ 1.2 trillion – mainly due to the weakening of the dollar, which made non-dollar loans translate to a larger dollar amount. The ratio of foreign debt to earnings from exports of goods and services, however, continued to decline for the fourth year since 1985 and stood in 1990 at 16% above its 1980 value (Table 1.2). Over US$ 40 billion was transferred from the heavily indebted countries to other countries during 1985, compared to a net positive inflow of approximately US$ 9 billion in 1980. Interest payments were also almost 50% higher than they were a decade before and equalled the growth in export earnings.

Slow and uneven progress has been achieved in recent years in debt and debt-service reductions owing to complex negotiation processes, the divergence of interests and approaches among creditors, and uncertainties about the adjustment efforts of some debtors. With a deteriorating economic environment in many developing countries, resolve and capacity for undertaking measures for structural adjustments and stabilization have weakened. The new initiatives and developments underlying various recent multilateral plans have been evolved to help debt-ridden developing countries to pursue their stabilization and reform policies with vigour; for example, the Toronto Terms announced in June 1988 were targeted on rescheduling the official debt of sub-Saharan Africa and 18 countries benefited; the Brady Plan launched in March 1989 was aimed at lowering the debt burden of 19 middle-income debtor countries with predominantly commercial debts; the Paris Club launched a new strategy of offering more favourable terms for lower middle-income countries and an overall "forgiveness" of official development assistance loans to sub-Saharan Africa; the Enterprise for the Americas initiative was announced by the United States in June 1990 to boost economic reform and development in Latin America, and the Trinidad and Tobago Terms, targeted at poor countries undergoing economic adjustment programmes, were launched by the United Kingdom in September 1990. While all these aid initiatives are laudable, one should not ignore the drying up of development finance in general, which might impossibly prolong the already protracted debt crisis. According to the *World Economic Survey* (1991) (*6*), a key policy requirement for developing countries would be to create an economic environment conducive to an improvement in saving and investment performance, with the developed countries providing these countries with better access to international markets, granting differential and more favourable treatment for their exports, and ensuring continuity in existing preferential trade and aid arrangements. If the international economic conditions and domestic political conditions allow, highly indebted countries might continue to carry their debt burden for another decade, but only at the cost of economic stagnation or decline, to the detriment of the principle of equity and the process of development.

Resource allocation patterns

Savings and consumption

The amount of GDP invested is a reflection of physical capital such as equipment and buildings. Long-term experience of many countries, especially of the newly industrialized ones, has shown that for sustainable growth, large investments are necessary, together with the ability to use them efficiently. The capacity to invest depends on the ability of countries to mobilize internal savings and to supplement them with external resources.

Table 1.3 gives estimated shares of domestic investment, national savings and external resources in GDP by major world economic regions, for 1985 and 1989. For both the developed market economies and developing countries as a whole there was an increase of about 1% in the share of gross domestic savings in GDP; this equalled the gross domestic investment in these groups of countries, which means that net transfer of resources was negligible or nil (*6*). Also, for a large number of debt-ridden developing countries, investment remained

throughout the 1980s at levels significantly below that reached in 1980. Investment was increased in developing countries when the adjustment process focused on reducing government consumption expenditure; this released domestic savings for productive investment. However, for low- and middle-income countries, increasing savings by restraining the levels of consumption had limited scope, because overall domestic savings had remained at a low level; in fact, the average savings rate in the least developed countries fell by half, from about 6% during 1970–1980 to 3% in the 1980s (*8*), which in absolute terms was much lower due to a fall in overall output. Savings efforts had to be supplemented by external resources, which were insufficient. A recent study has shown that there was a global shortage of savings if one considered the total global surplus and total global deficit in countries' domestic budgets (Fig. 1.2). While the level of overall consumption may not be reducible in all cases, it should be possible to generate additional savings through a reallocation of consumption by reducing misdirected consumption (e.g., military spending) and by encouraging a shift from inefficient production enterprises. However, such a shift requires fundamental changes in the political underpinnings of society: a new "development ethic" that binds together "social groups in a winning ground coalition" would have to be considered (*9*). This would be a time-consuming process. Also, since there are strong reasons to support the view that it is not savings that cause investment but investment that produces growth and savings, it was becoming increasingly necessary to review allocation patterns and raise savings, possibly through a major reorientation of tax expenditures (*5*).

Central government expenditure and disarmament

When saving is impossible, other options available through a reallocation of government expenditure must be considered. Table 1.4

Table 1.3

Investment, savings, and net transfers as percentage of GDP: developing countries, 1980, 1985, and 1989

Country groupings	Gross domestic investment			Gross domestic savings			Net transfers of resources		
	1980	1985	1989	1980	1985	1989	1980	1985	1989
All developing countries	25.2	23.2	24.7	26.6	23.6	24.7	−1.4	−0.4	...
of which, 15 heavily indebted countries	23.9	16.4	19.5	23.4	21.2	21.6	0.5	−4.8	1.8

Source: United Nations (1991) and reference (*6*).

shows the percentage of central government expenditure on defence, education, and health in different regions of the world for 1983 and for the latest available year. These figures are difficult to compare across regions because in many large economies, such as the Federal Republic of Germany, India, and the United States, states and local authorities account for much general government revenue and are responsible for government functions such as education and health; defence, however, is invariably with the central government. The overall impression remains that defence takes a large share of central government expenditure, and the proportion spent on the health sector in the developing countries seems to have been about 4% during 1983 and 1988 (with no reduction except in Asia). After the mid-1980s, military expenditure in real terms in both the developed and the developing countries stabilized and then declined, and the declining trend in global military expenditure continued into 1989 (*6*).

The waning threat of war between the largest nuclear powers provides an opportunity for realizing a peaceful world. While some costs would be incurred in the short and medium terms for verification and related activities, there was an anticipation that a substantial reduction in military expenditure could constitute a major new source of resources for investments in human development and physical infrastructure, to enable the world to achieve a higher living standard. However, for the "peace dividend" hoped for in the late 1980s to materialize, a durable peace and a world in which disputes are solved not by armed force but through negotiations will be necessary. Until then, significant additional resources even for health, might not be forthcoming, even when badly needed.

Fig. 1.2

Global supply of and demand for funds (based on current account balance)

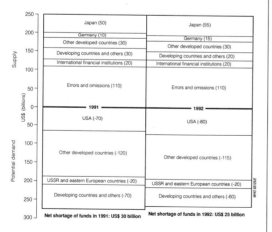

Transfers of cooperation funds for the Gulf are excluded in current account balance for 1991.
Source: Japan Institute for Information on International Finance

Table 1.4
Percentage of central government spending on defence, education, and health, 1983 and latest available year

		Defence	Education	Health
World	1983	15.5	5.0	9.7
	1987	16.0	4.8	11.0
Developed market economies	1983	15.9	3.8	11.1
	1987	16.7	3.5	12.6
of which, United States	1983	23.7	1.9	10.6
	1989	24.6	1.8	12.9
Developing countries	1983	13.9	9.7	3.9
	1988	13.1	10.6	4.0
of which, Europe	1983	20.3	4.9	1.3
	1989	22.1	6.6	2.6
Asia	1983	20.7	9.9	2.9
	1989	16.9	9.7	2.5
Africa	1983	11.1	11.3	3.4
	1985	10.3	12.4	3.9
Latin America	1983	5.5	9.2	4.9
	1988	5.7	9.7	5.0
Middle East	1983	17.0	11.9	5.0
	1988	18.3	16.1	5.8

Source: United Nations (1991) and reference (*6*).

Poverty and social justice

During the 1980s, there has been some increase in production and disposable income in some regions but stagnation in others. The overall inequalities in income distribution among countries remain extremely large. Recent studies by the World Bank, the United Nations, and OECD have reported a significant drop in the *proportion* of people living below the poverty line between 1970 and 1985; the *number* of people living in poverty, however, increased substantially during the period because of the rapid growth in population. The studies also show that the 1980s – often called a "lost decade" for the poor – did not, in fact, reverse the overall trend of progress; the incomes of most of the world's poor were rising, with improvements in under-5 mortality, primary school enrolment ratio, and other social indicators (*10*). However, the burden of poverty has been spread unevenly – among the regions of the developing world, among countries within those regions, and among population groups and localities within countries, particularly with an upsurge in urban slums. Except in Latin America, the poor are more numerous in rural than in urban areas. In a number of low- and middle-income countries, particularly in Africa, large segments of the population continue to live in conditions of absolute poverty. To them the quinquennium 1985–90 has brought little relief.

A survey of development strategies in some countries of south Asia has also shown that during the last four decades, national income has increased but the extent of absolute poverty has not diminished. Increased food output had no significant effect on the nutritional status of the poor, mainly due to increase in population and unequal income distribution. This is partly ascribed to government spending on social and health services being ineffective in benefiting the poor. The health status of the poor segments of the population continued to remain low even when the overall availability of health facilities was improving. In India, most of the second- and third-level care as well as private practitioners were in urban areas. Yet the infant mortality rate continued to be substantially higher in urban slums than in rural areas. It has also been claimed that this situation could be a result of the current development strategy; the existing strategies for economic growth might be perpetuating poverty among the majority of people. Such a situation would call for innovative approaches, and several alternatives have been proposed and tested. As an example, a poverty alleviation programme in Sri Lanka considered human beings as the primary resource and stressed self-reliance and sustainability as well as social and cultural acceptability. With appropriate policy interventions concerned with the social dimensions of adjustment and directed to the poor and vulnerable populations, it was possible to achieve a maximum rate of poverty reduction without causing at the same time distortions in economic mechanisms that were set in motion to accelerate growth in production and employment (10,11). It is still anticipated that development policies will be readjusted and that, between 1985 and 2000, the prevalence of poverty in the developing world might be reduced from 33% to 18% and the number of poor from 1100 million to 825 million.

Implications for health

The prospects for global economic growth in the near future have deteriorated with the continued decline in per capita output in many economies – e.g., those in transition (eastern Europe and the USSR) and those disrupted by the crisis in the Middle East. Weaker growth is expected in both developing and developed countries, and growth in per capita output may be negligible or even negative for many of the least developed countries, particularly in sub-Saharan Africa. Efforts to increase earnings through trade may not be very successful either, in view of the protectionist tendencies in individual countries and the substitution of unilateral action for multilateral approaches to resolve trade problems. There is also uncertainty over the eventual outcome of the Uruguay round of multilateral trade negotiations. With trade becoming one of the more dynamic elements in the world economy and given the above uncertainties and constraints, the increased availability of net resources for domestic use cannot be relied upon.

With respect to the international flow of financial resources to developing countries, the prospects are not bright in a world that is short of capital and faces new demands to finance the economic transition in central and eastern Europe. There will not be any significant additional external resources for the developing countries in general and the least developed countries in particular to accelerate their development activities unless appropriate steps are taken concerning trade and international aid policies. Already it is being realized that the situation can be improved if both developed and developing countries give renewed attention to the appropriate policies (domestic and international) for expanding the flow of development finance in the years ahead.

There is an increasing recognition at the international level that institutional changes, social welfare policies targeted at vulnerable population groups and priority areas such as nutrition, and measures to make income distribution less unequal can have a much greater impact on social welfare and social progress than an expansion in output (11). In choosing an approach to human resource and institutional development in accordance with national priorities, values, traditions, customs, and stage of development, special attention has to be given to education and health; they are essential aspects of human resource development (*12*). At the special session of the United Nations devoted to International Cooperation in April 1990 (*2*), considerable agreement was reached on the fundamental goals and strategies for the Fourth Development Decade and also on major international economic policy questions. At the start of the 1990s, the General Assembly saw an "opportunity to restore a long-term approach to development", moving beyond short-term adjustments and focusing on the primary objective of the betterment of the human condition by responding to the needs of and maximizing the potential of all members of society. Fresh approaches to the formulation and implementation of health, nutrition, housing, population, and other social welfare policies as a key to both improving individual welfare and successful development have been called for at national and international levels.

Emphasis on the social and political dimensions of development – poverty alleviation, social justice, civil liberties, etc. – is receiving more attention from international development organizations and agencies. UNDP and the World Bank, for example, are now going back to their approach and perspective of the 1960s and 1970s, when the United Nations studied and searched for a unified approach to development, and are again stressing the positive implications of a socially responsible development strategy for developing and developed countries alike (*13*). Policies focusing on "investing in people" as a powerful engine for development are being promoted (*14*). In such an environment, the role of national policies also requires review and revision. With the shrinking in the global availability of external resources for transfer to needy countries, it becomes necessary to make judicious use of available national resources and to adopt policies and strategies that can improve or maintain growth (*6*).

Past trends indicate that the percentage of central government spending for health has in fact increased in both developed market economies and in developing countries. Recent studies by UNESCO and the United Nations have also shown that relatively speaking the health sector has been enjoying an increase in the proportion of central government expenditure devoted to health during the 1980s while that on education has been falling; central governments seem to favour health spending rather than education (*6,15*). This is a reversal of trends observed in the 1960s, when the preferential order of social aims was nutrition, education, and health (*16*). It is increasingly recognized that health is basic to human development, and investment in people must be made with special attention to health improvement. Perhaps the health sector is becoming more vocal in claiming and getting its share in government spending. It is clear, however, that, with severe constraints on external and internal resources, the chances are poor for an increase in allocation for the health sector.

The health sector is preparing itself for this eventuality and has become prudent in making the best use of available resources by cutting down misdirected allocation, by sharpening priorities, and by implementing policies and strategies that improve effectiveness and reduce waste. Health authorities are also putting stress on the development of "healthy policies" in general; on discouraging smoking through pricing, education, and agricultural policies rather than secondary prevention for cancer patients; on promotion of safe traffic through "healthy road" policies rather than emergency wards and rehabilitation centres. The issue being addressed is not so much that of getting more money for health – it is rather that of spending more judiciously the resources already available.

Demographic trends

Health, population, and development are inextricably intertwined. Social development, for example, requires higher educational levels for women, one of the principal underlying factors in improving child health and survival. Economic development is generally associated with large population displacements towards urban areas as the foci of economic growth. Cities are more than economic powerhouses; they are social and cultural centres, and each city has its unique character and sense of place. Urbanization can provide more employment opportunities, better education, better housing, better nutrition, better access to health services, all of which contribute to better health. Attempts to slow urbanization by rural development schemes have sometimes been based on the false assumption that the rural and urban spheres are separate and self-contained, and not an interdependent whole. However, rapid urbanization in developing countries can bring with it a large burden of disease and premature death caused by deficiencies in housing, roads, safe water, sanitation, and basic health and environmental services.

In a situation of limited resources for health, when the demand for services will always exceed supply, the optimum allocation of these resources is closely dependent on the demographic situation as well as changes in it over time. Thus the size of the population, its sex and age structure, and its geographical distribution, as well as rates of change in these variables, have significant implications for health services. Trends in fertility and to a lesser extent migration exert an impact on the health status of a population (for example, shorter birth intervals tend to decrease child survival). Similarly, demographic trends such as rapid population aging have a major impact on the need for specific health and social services for the elderly. High fertility and uncontrolled population migration may also have serious negative consequences for social and economic development.

Population size and growth rates

Between 1985 and 1990, the estimated population of the world grew from 4851 million to 5292 million, or by about 9%. The number of people living in the developing countries of the world in 1990 was 4056 million, of whom almost 450 million were living in the least developed countries. In contrast, about 1220 million or about 23% of the world's population were living in the developed world. In 1990, ten countries had a population in excess of 100 million. The two most populous countries, China and India, together account for 2000 million people or 50% of the total population of the developing world. Other developing countries with populations in excess of 100 million in 1990 include Indonesia (184 million), Brazil (150 million), Pakistan (123 million), Bangladesh (116 million), and Nigeria (109 million). Mexico, with a population of 89 million in 1990, can also be expected to reach 100 million during the 1990s (17).

Globally, world population growth is slowing from an annual rate of increase of 2.1% in the late 1960s to about 1.7% today. Growth rates are expected to continue their decline to reach an annual average rate of population increase of about 1% by about 2020. Population growth is still considerably higher in the developing world (2.1% per year between 1985 and 1990) compared with the developed countries (0.6% per year). The average rate of population increase for the least developed countries over the last 5 years was 2.8% per year.

This deceleration in population growth is also reflected in the progression towards replacement-level fertility (i.e., a net reproduction rate of 1.00, this rate indicating the extent to which the current generation of women of childbearing age will replace themselves). Globally, the net reproduction rate is expected to reach replacement level in about 2025. For the developed countries, replacement-level fertility was achieved in the mid-1970s whereas for the developing countries, the net reproduction rate is currently still about 1.6 female children per woman and is expected to decline by 2020-2025 to about 1.06 female children per woman, or just above replacement level. For the least developed countries, the net reproduction rate is still in excess of 2.2 per woman and is projected to be 1.3 in 2020–2025.

In the absence of significant net migration, population growth reflects the excess of fertility over mortality rates. Changes in the crude birth and death rates between 1985 and 1990 can be seen from Table 1.5. Fertility levels, as might be expected, have changed very little over this period. Birth rates remain three times higher for the least developed countries than for the developed countries. Much the same picture emerges from an examination of trends in the total fertility rate (average number of births per woman); on average, a woman in the least developed countries can expect to give birth to 6.1 children in her lifetime, compared with 1.8 in the developed market economies and 3.8 for the developing world as a whole.

The stability of crude death rates is also evident from Table 1.5, with no significant changes between 1985 and 1990. Comparisons of the *level* of mortality using the crude death rate can be misleading, however, owing to the fact that populations in which a high proportion of people survive to the older ages have comparatively more deaths. Thus the crude death rate for the developed market economies is identical to that for the developing countries as a whole. Measures of mortality that take into account age composition, such as life expectancy at birth,

are thus more relevant indicators of health condition.

These increases in population have led to higher population densities, particularly in south-east Asia. Between 1985 and 1990, the population per square kilometre increased from 24 to 28 in the least developed countries and from 47 to 52 in the developing countries as a whole, i.e., more than 10%. Population density in the developed countries, on the other hand, has remained relatively stable at around 20 persons per square kilometre.

Sex and age composition

The relative numbers of males and females in a population reflects the cumulative impact of differential mortality and migration on the sex ratio at birth. Short-term changes in these determinants are unlikely and so the population sex ratio has not changed markedly since 1985. There are 4% more males than females in the developing world as a whole whereas in the developed countries, where differential mortality strongly favours females, females outnumber males by about 6%. This is particularly evident in the countries of eastern Europe, where there are about 91 males for every 100 females.

Of much greater significance for health and social policy is the age composition of the population, given the marked age-dependent demand for services. Increasing numbers of the elderly

Table 1.5
Trends in fertility and mortality, 1985 to 1990

Country groupings	Crude birth rate		Crude death rate		Total fertility rate		Life expectancy for both sexes	
	1985	1990	1985	1990	1985	1990	1985	1990
Developing countries	31.3	30.4	10.2	9.4	4.1	3.8	61.0	62.8
of which, least developed	45.1	44.3	17.4	15.8	6.3	6.1	48.5	50.7
Eastern Europe	17.8	16.7	10.8	10.4	2.3	2.2	69.5	71.0
Developed market economies	14.2	13.8	9.2	9.3	1.8	1.8	74.9	75.8

will obviously place greater demands on pensions and social security systems in countries where these are common, in addition to the demands on the health sector itself. Studies in Europe and North America have found that the elderly typically account for 30–40% of bed-days in hospitals and of visits to general practitioners, quite disproportionate to their share of the population. "Disability" services will also be increasingly demanded by the elderly since the evidence suggests that the recent gains in life expectancy enjoyed by the aged have not been disability-free. Therefore, increasing attention should be given to maintaining the elderly in good health through promotive and preventive action. Social and tax policies must also be developed to strengthen families and local communities which are in reality the main providers of care and support for the elderly. Health and social services will also need to take into account the fact that future elderly populations will be better educated and thus more likely to demand more care, higher quality care, and often more individual care. Again, the demographic processes (fertility, mortality, migration) which determine population age structure are relatively invariant over short time periods, and hence there has been comparatively little change in age structure since 1985. There have been some significant trends, however. The continued decline in mortality in the developed market-economy countries has led to a further increase, from 12.0% to 12.8%, in the proportion of the population of these countries aged 65 and over. Although in the developing countries the proportion aged 65 and over has changed only marginally, from 4.2% to 4.5%, the numbers of elderly have risen dramatically from 153 million in 1985 to 182 million in 1990 and now exceed the elderly population (145 million) in the developed countries. Moreover, this differential is expected to continue to widen so that by the year 2000, the number of people aged 65 and over in developing countries is projected to reach 250 million, or almost 50% more than the 173 million projected for the developed world. At the younger ages, only about one-fifth of the population of the developed market economies (one-quarter of the population in eastern Europe) is under the age of 15 years, compared with 45% in the least developed countries.

An alternative view of changes in age composition of the population can be obtained from population dependency ratios, which give the population aged 0–14 and/or 65 years and over per 100 population aged 15–64. In other words, these ratios summarize the size and nature of the population dependent on the working-age population. In 1990, there were on average 17.9 persons aged 65 and over per 100 population of working-age in the developed countries, compared with 17.1/100 in 1985. This elderly dependency ratio is more than twice that of the developing countries as a whole (7.4/100).

Conversely, the child dependency ratio is substantially higher in the developing countries (59.2/100) compared to developed countries (32.9/100) and reaching 84.7 per 100 in the least developed countries. That is, there is almost one child per adult of working age in the least developed countries compared with one for every three adults in the developed world. There has been relatively little change in the ratio since 1985.

Urbanization

In 1990, an estimated 2400 million or 45% of the world's population lived in urban areas: 37% of the population of developing regions (1500 million) and 73% (900 million) of the developed world. During 1985–1990, the urban population growth rate was 3.1% per year for the world (4.5% in the developing countries and 0.8% in the developed countries). According to United Nations estimates, the rate of urban population growth peaked in 1980–1985 at 4.6% per year for the developing world and is now declining (18). None the less, it is clear that the developing regions are undergoing rapid urbanization, and this is projected to continue for decades to come. Thus, between 1990 and 2025, the total urban population in developing regions is projected to increase threefold to 4000 million, or 61% of the population.

Nearly two-thirds of the urban population of the developing world live in Asia. A further 20% of the total live in Latin America and one in seven in Africa. The least developed countries are also the least urbanized with only about 20% of the population living in urban areas, although this proportion is expected to more than double to 44% by 2025. Conversely, about 73% of the population of the developed world in 1990 lived in urban areas, slightly more than the 72% estimated for 1985.

Continued rapid population growth and the pervasive spread of poverty, particularly in developing countries, are straining society's capacity to provide environmental health facilities and services. In many developing countries with massive growth of the urban population, the degradation of living conditions is of crisis proportions. In both urban and rural areas, a large burden of diseases and premature death is caused by deficiencies in housing, roads, piped water, sanitation drainage, electricity, and basic health and environmental services.

The health of residents of low-quality housing in urban areas is adversely influenced firstly by poverty and its associated limited education, insufficient diet, overcrowding, and lack of health care or protection; secondly by deficiencies in the built environment and basic sanitation, together with the hazards of pollution and traffic; and thirdly by social and psychosocial instability and insecurity, which cause stress and alienation. UNEP estimates that overall about one-third of the urban population in the developing world live in such conditions (*19*).

What is particularly important about this process from the health viewpoint is the fact that the urbanization process in developing countries will imply a much greater number of "megacities", i.e., cities with 10 million or more inhabitants (Fig. 1.3). This growth will increase the demands on health and social services, especially for the urban poor, and may thus exacerbate differentials in health status between different population subgroups within these large urban agglomerations. Social disintegration and problems of management are frequent in such human settlements, as shown by violence, drug abuse and the collapse of public services. On the other hand, the number of cities with more than 10 million population in the developed world is expected to increase at a much slower pace, and will be substantially less than in developing countries by the year 2000.

Case studies in some cities have confirmed that those living in poorer districts have much poorer health status than wealthier urban residents; infant and child mortality rates are typically three to five times higher among the urban poor[1] and often exceed the rates in rural areas. Malnutrition, diarrhoeal disease, food poisoning, and pneumonia have been found to be markedly higher among the urban poor compared with wealthier areas of cities in Asia and Latin America. A lack of readily available drinking-water, of sewerage connections or other systems to dispose of human wastes, of garbage disposal and of basic measures to prevent disease ensures that many life-threatening conditions are endemic among the urban poor.

None the less, the relative dearth of disaggregated health information for different population subgroups within major urban agglomerations is a major obstacle to identifying the priority health problems adequately and thus to defining intersectoral policies and strategies designed to reduce what are undoubtedly substantial intra-urban differentials in health status and social services in major urban agglomerations throughout the world.

---

1. A study in India found a tenfold difference in infant mortality rates between the richest and poorest families in some cities.

Fig. 1.3
Cities having more than 10 million inhabitants in 1990

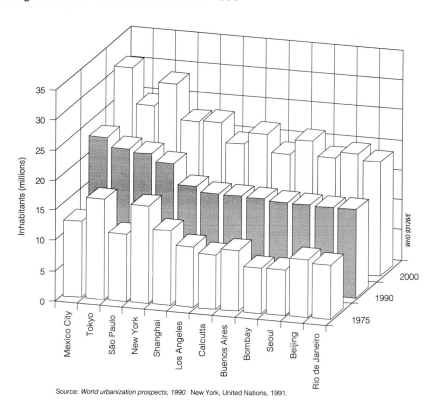

Source: *World urbanization prospects, 1990.* New York, United Nations, 1991.

International migration (*20*)

The late 1980s witnessed the resurgence of international migration as an important demographic phenomenon, especially for countries in which low rates of natural increase prevail. The general relaxation of travel and emigration regulations in the countries of eastern Europe that has accompanied the political and economic changes taking place in the region has led to important migrant outflows of asylum-seekers in other European countries. In addition, efficient and cheap transport coupled with the proliferation of regional conflict has contributed to increasing the presence of asylum-seekers from developing countries in the developed world. Although the recent events in western Asia have already changed drastically the migration dynamics in the region, by the late 1980s the member states of the Gulf Cooperation Council were hosting a very sizeable foreign population, estimated at 7.2 million in 1985. Evidence from the main labour-exporting countries of south and south-east Asia suggests that the inflow of migrant workers to western Asia declined during the late 1980s, a trend that is likely to be exacerbated by the conflict now affecting the region. Almost no new information is available on non-refugee migration in Africa and Latin America. Globally, the number of refugees increased by about 70% during the 1980s, rising from 8.5 million in 1980 to 14.5 in 1989.

Though most countries perceive the level of immigration and emigration in their countries as satisfactory, concerns over immigration are most widespread in Europe. Surveys indicate that many of the European countries view immigration levels as excessive and almost one in two European countries intend to reduce the level. A growing concern has been illegal immigration. With the stabilization of the foreign populations legally present in most western European countries, policy measures are now directed towards integration. The presence of significant numbers of foreigners has prompted adverse reactions and a rise in xenophobia in some countries.

In the African region, which is by no means a homogeneous entity, international migration policies vary greatly between the major labour-sending and labour-receiving countries. Countries that attract foreign labour are more often concerned about the influx of undocumented migrants. Some 15% of Latin American countries seek to increase immigration, but economic stagnation and political conditions made some of them less attractive for permanent settlement and more likely to experience emigration, particularly of skilled workers, to the USA or Europe. In addition, emigration to southern Europe, particularly to Italy and Spain, has become more attractive for people in North Africa, and the prospect of free movement within the European Community acts as a magnet.

In Asia, government intervention in the regulation of international migration is common: relatively few countries in the region report no intervention with respect to either immigration or emigration. Immigration is often perceived as too high by the oil-producing countries of western Asia, and policies to reduce immigration are widespread. On the other hand, emigration is viewed as too low by major labour-sending countries such as Bangladesh, Indonesia, Jordan, Pakistan, and Turkey, most of whom seek to increase it. In Oceania, governments generally perceive both immigration and emigration levels as satisfactory, and maintaining them stable is their most common goal. A few countries in that region have taken specific measures to control migration.

Social trends

It is difficult to obtain from existing data a precise notion of social changes globally over the period 1985–1990 as regards destitution, hunger, deficient housing, or ill-health, but the global indicators used in this section do convey a sense of the direction and magnitude of selected aspects, such as food supply, education, the use of the media, or employment. In general, trends were positive.

Food consumption and security

The Committee for World Food Security of FAO reported at its 16th session a record production of 1779 million tons of cereals in the world in 1990, 4% higher than the previous year, and in excess of estimated consumption. At the same time, the report confirmed that cereal production had declined in Africa and Latin America. The Director-General of FAO launched an appeal for aid to 24 countries with food deficits.

The report reflects the food situation during the 1980s: a sufficiency in production in the world as a whole combined with serious deficits in individual regions and in countries within regions. According to FAO reports (21), severe and increasing food supply problems were reported from large parts of sub-Saharan Africa. To avert widespread famine, massive and sustained international assistance would be required in 1991 in at least two countries, the situation would remain critical in three others, and had deteriorated in several Sahelian countries following poor harvests in 1990.

Access to food was reported to have deteriorated in several countries in South America where cereal stocks had been drawn down sharply after three successive years of declining output. Recent developments in central and eastern Europe and in the Middle East have added a new element of uncertainty to the world food situation. Food systems have also been seriously disturbed in a number of countries, particularly in Africa, by military conflict. The result there may be famine or near-famine. Elsewhere, problems are exacerbated by the lack of transport to ship food from areas with a food surplus to areas with a food deficit.

National food deficits are made good in part by imports which, however, many countries find it increasingly difficult to finance, and to a smaller degree by food aid. Much of the widespread malnutrition in the world today is the result of poverty. A large number of people simply lack the means to buy sufficient or appropriate food. Just how many people are malnourished or hungry is not known with certainty, however. "The World Food Council estimated about 1000 million people were chronically hungry in the mid-1980s. FAO and the World Bank gave somewhat more conservative figures. The Bank estimated that in 1980 about one-third of the world's population, some 740 million people in 87 developing countries (excluding China) did not consume enough calories for an active working life. ... FAO, using a more rigorous criterion ... estimated 325 million undernourished people in 1979–1981 in 98 'developing market economies'" (22). Problems of hunger, linked to poverty, exist also in the developed countries although on a smaller scale. Other problems there are the result of overconsumption in general and of fat in particular, resulting in disease associated with such excess.

There is a wide gap in food supply between regions. Africa has the lowest calorie supply per capita, North America and Europe (east and west) the highest by a very large margin. In 1983–1985, requirements as estimated by FAO and WHO failed to be met in 28 out of 139 countries (ignoring minor deviations, of 5% or less), 16 of them in Africa (23).

There have been dramatic improvements in some countries, as in China, stability or a modest improvement in most others. With the exception of Africa, all regions increased their supply of calories, but some considerably more so than others. The centrally planned economies of Asia

(mainly China), the Middle East (e.g., Jordan, Libyan Arab Jamahiriya, Saudi Arabia) and North America (Canada and the USA) did best, Africa and the Far East worst. Within the Far East (which, as defined by FAO, includes southern Asia) Indonesia fared better than others. On the whole, however, and with the notable exception of China, the regions with the lowest levels of calorie supply tended to maintain their position to the end of the decade.

The supply of protein changed in much the same way. Substantial gains were recorded in China, North America, and Europe, a substantial loss in Africa. Nor has excess consumption abated in the developed countries. The supply of per capita calories increased by a further 3% between 1979–1981 and 1986–1988, while the supply of fat rose by no less than 6%.

Education

There has been steady improvement. School enrolment rates increased over the period 1985–1990 in all the world's regions and for each of the three age-groups to reach for the world as a whole an estimated 80% for the 6–11-year age-group, 55% at secondary level (ages 12–17) and 20% for the tertiary level age-group, 18–23 (24). The level of education attained may be a more relevant indicator than school enrolment, but virtually no comparable data exist of changes in attainment over the period.

The global figures conceal considerable variation, however. In non-Arab African countries primary-age enrolment made little headway against the surge of population, and the level remained at about 50%. While females continue to have less access than males, the gap between males and females narrowed over the period in most of the world's regions as regards primary, but much less so as regards secondary and tertiary, enrolment. Thus in the Arab states, where females have been particularly disadvantaged, the gap in enrolment for primary education narrowed from 17% to 14%, but by only from 18% to 16% for secondary education. In Africa (excluding Arab states), the gap actually widened at the tertiary level from 7 to about 9 percentage points.

Adult literacy has similarly shown improvement over the period (Fig. 1.4 and box). The proportion of illiterate adults has been declining for some years, but for the first time since statistics became available, the absolute number of such illiterates in the world also declined between 1985 and 1990, namely from 949.5 to 948.1 million (the difference may be the result of different estimation methods, but the trend is probably significant) (24).

The proportions of literate persons increased in each region, for both men and women. The increase in percentage points between 1985 and 1990 was greater for men than for women, though from higher initial levels. It was greater also in Africa than in the other regions.

Numerous studies have shown the clear relationship between the ability to read and write, the practice of family planning, and falling infant mortality. Illiteracy, especially among women, thus continued to be a serious obstacle to health development. Closer contacts between ministries of education and health would be needed to develop mutually supportive education and health policies.

Communications

While education, including the ability to read, is clearly important to health, it is no longer the only means of conveying information. Radio and television have become important means of communication.[1]

---

1. Communications in a wider sense are facilitated also by the construction of roads, better means of transport (on which however no relevant global data are available), and by the concentration of the population in towns, where in many cases they can be much more readily reached with health care or health information than in scattered rural areas.

Global indicator 11
The adult literacy rate, by sex, in all identifiable subgroups

Fig. 1.4
Average adult literacy rates for countries in various stages of development (global indicator 11), 1985 and 1991

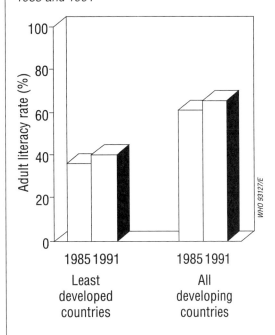

There has been a significant increase in the use of television in both the developed countries, where near saturation has been reached with one receiver for every two people, and in developing countries, where the ratio doubled between 1980 and 1985. However, even in 1988 there was only one set for every 22 people in the world, and only one for about 70 people in Africa (excluding Arab states) (24).

The possible impact on health of the media depends also on programme content. UNESCO has given some details for a number of countries. Thus informative, cultural, and educational programmes, which may have a bearing on health education, typically use up a little more than half the broadcasting time. There is, however, considerable variation among countries – in Africa from about 72% to 35%, in Asia from 90% to 15%.

The number of radios increased in all the regions more rapidly during the 1980s than the number of television receivers. Even Africa, least well supplied, had by 1988 one receiver for every seven people. Newspaper circulation also increased slightly, by about 2% for the world as a whole, but by about 30% for the developing countries as a group from a relatively low base (*24*). Mass media are an important resource of health promotion and health education. However, collaboration between the health sector and the mass media is not well established in many countries, and lack of mutual understanding between media and health workers is still common. The trend is towards better coordination, thus aiming for a more effective impact of media on health.

Employment and unemployment

Major structural changes in employment and unemployment are likely to have a bearing on health. Some of the significant features in recent years have been (1) changes in participation rates in the labour force, particularly of women; (2) the sharp decline, absolute in some regions, relative in others, of the proportion of the economically active in agriculture; (3) a continued upward trend in international migration of labour; and (4) changes in the nature of youth unemployment, especially in developed countries.

As shown by the International Labour Organisation, labour force participation rates (the employed plus the unemployed as a percentage of the population aged 10 and over) of the younger age group (10–19) and the older age group (65 and over) have declined considerably in both developed and developing countries, and for men as well as women (*25*).

On the other hand, the remarkable growth in the employment of women aged between 20 and 64, particularly in the developed countries, came to a halt around 1980. The developing regions vary greatly as regards women's participation in the labour force. In many countries of east Asia and Latin America, participation rates increased considerably from 1950, whereas they remained stagnant or declined in Africa and in parts of south Asia.

The composition of the three main sectors of employment changed sharply between 1950 and 1980 (and on what evidence there is, continued to do so from 1980 to 1990): in the developed countries a decline in agriculture and secondary industry into tertiary activities; in many developing countries a decline in agriculture into secondary and, depending on the region, increasingly into tertiary sectors (*25*).

Apart from these broad structural shifts, significant changes are taking place within each major sector as regards techniques, materials and product. Examples are the shift from subsistence to cash crops in agriculture, towards computerized processing in the service sectors, and away from asbestos in the construction industry. Some of the implications for health are well documented (as for asbestos), while others remain controversial – for example, the impact on nutrition, and thereby on health, of the shift to cash crops.

Although it is often said that, globally, capital is more mobile than labour, a large number of people seek employment outside their own country. The problems of such migrants, including their need for health care, have been well documented by the International Labour Organisation (*26*) and have been mentioned on pages 26 and 27. Reliable data on migrant workers are sparse, particularly on the many illegal migrants. The number of migrant workers in the early 1980s is estimated at between 20 and 22 million, including between 5 and 7 million workers from developing countries in northern America, between 6 and 7 million in western Europe, 3 million in western Asia, and 3 to 4 million in Latin America. Numbers have increased since 1980 in the few countries or regions for which data are available. For example, the Federal Republic of Germany reported an annual inflow of 95 000 migrants in 1985, but ten times this number in 1989, the great majority from eastern European countries including the former German Democratic Republic. In the Middle East, the number of legal foreign nationals had increased from 2.8 million in 1975 to 7.2 million in 1985, but declined after 1985 to about 6.3 million in 1989, and more dramatically as the result of the crisis in the Middle East in 1990. Until 1990, the number of illegal workers is said to have increased sharply in some Middle East countries (27).

Unemployment figures are more complete in the developed countries than in most of the developing countries, in which in any case the concept may be largely inappropriate. It is likely, however, that in the course of adjustment recruitment opportunities in urban areas of Africa and Latin America have stagnated while the number of candidates has increased with demographic pressure.

In western Europe and the USA, unemployment declined during the second half of the 1980s but has continued to be a major preoccupation. Many of the unemployed in the developed countries are young people. Several new features of youth unemployment have emerged during the second half of the 1980s: (1) more unemployment among disadvantaged young people, and a longer duration of unemployment than before; (2) even the better educated and trained have considerable difficulty in finding secure jobs; (3) labour force participation rates have dropped for young people while educational enrolment has risen; (4) there is now a problem of providing opportunities for the "high risk" generation of young people born between the 1950s and mid 1960s, for whom there are relatively few jobs. It is in this group that problems of drug dependency or crime are frequent.

Studies in a number of countries have documented severe negative effects on health among unemployed persons and preventive action would seem to need strengthening. The special problems of migrant workers have also received increased attention. These include malnutrition, social and cultural isolation, work accidents, and problems from lack of understanding of the language spoken in the recipient country.

Women and development

Considerable interest in women and development has been stimulated both by the United Nations Decade for Women (1976–1985) and by the promotion of primary health care, which together form the link between women's health and overall progress in health and development. Today, the significance of women's health and socioeconomic well-being is not only increasingly recognized but is seen as a necessity for sustainable development.

Some of the positive outcomes of the last decade were: the inclusion of women's needs, and gender responsiveness, on the agendas of governments, agencies, and nongovernmental organizations; changes in legislation and development policies; the establishment of mechanisms at various levels concerned with women and development; and problem identification supported by an improving information base. Initial indifference to acknowledging, promoting, and enhancing women's role in development began to give way to support for specific programmes aimed at redressing some of the consequences suffered by women in the process of social and economic change. These efforts helped to further women's rights and to encourage data-gathering, but did not lead to the large-scale integration of women into development. Despite some positive results it has become clear that overall progress has been slow and patchy. Even in developed countries the substantial gains achieved by women have had their limitations.

Reflection of the above factors in the area of women and development can be noted in the indicators of health of women as a continuum over their life span. In most human populations, the average expectation of life at birth, an indicator of health conditions, is higher for women than men. However, there are marked differences among countries. In the developed countries, during the period 1985–1990, women live about seven years longer than men; in the developing countries they live only three years longer. Over time, the gap has tended to increase in developing countries, where there is substantially greater room for improving health conditions.

The health of women in the years from 15 to 45 is predominantly influenced by their reproductive and maternal roles. In most parts of the world women spend most of this period either pregnant or breast-feeding. Their health during this period influences their long-term health and that of other family members, especially their children. Of crucial importance is the ability to control their fertility through access to socioculturally acceptable family planning information and services, which, for most women, in addition to preserving their health, is a prerequisite for equitable participation in development. The health effects of reproduction are reflected in patterns of mortality. In many developing countries as many as half the deaths of women of reproductive age are due to pregnancy-related causes. Each year, about half a million women die from causes related to pregnancy and childbirth. All but 6000 of these deaths take place in developing countries, which account for 99% of all maternal deaths. Other health issues of prime importance include infertility, infections of the reproductive tract, sexually transmitted diseases, AIDS, and cancers of the reproductive system. In developed countries, although health care is accessible to most women, there is a growing concern about the over-use of sophisticated technologies, particularly in pregnancy and childbirth.

There has been much progress over the past three decades in providing education facilities for women. Yet there were about 950 million illiterate people in 1985 compared with 890 million in 1970. Women accounted for 60% of the total in 1985. In the developed countries, in 1985, the proportion of women who were illiterate was 2.6% while the corresponding figure for men was 1.7%. In contrast, in the developing countries of Africa, 64.5% of women and 43.3% of men were illiterate; in Asia, the corresponding figures were 47.4% and 25.6%; and in Latin America 19.2% and 15.3%. Inequalities in literacy and other education achievements are a direct result of social or family attitudes and unequal access to educational institutions.

There are marked variations among countries in the share of women in the labour force. In the centrally planned economies, the share of women in the labour force in 1985 was nearly half of the total labour force. In developed market economies, the corresponding proportion was 40%. Among developed market economy countries, the share of women was particularly high in North America (41%). Among developing countries in 1985, the highest female share was 43% in China. This figure compares with 28% in other Asian countries. The female share in Africa was 35% and in Latin America and the Caribbean 27% in the same year. There is also a substantial gap in earnings between men and women, with female workers receiving lower wages than male workers, but the earning differentials between male and female employees vary greatly from country to country.

Women's contribution to the formal health care system is well recognized, and in nearly every country, regardless of the level of social and economic development, the majority of health workers are women – i.e., primary health care workers, nurses, midwives, laboratory and research workers, doctors, and many other categories. The proportion of female doctors ranges from 3% to 30% in developing countries and from 8% to 70% in developed countries, although globally the numbers of women graduating each year have increased from a quarter to a third of the total over the past decade. However, very few women doctors hold positions of authority, even in those countries where women make up the majority of doctors.

For these reasons, among others, the poor condition of women with regard to health and development generally persists or has deteriorated, though it is no longer seen as trivial or "merely" a result of prejudice, inequity, and injustice, but as a major contributor to ineffective development. The challenge now lies in finding the best means to integrate women effectively and fully in the development process. In the 1990s the approaches to women's concerns will need to shift from the sidelines of development to a concerted initiative to bring women into the mainstream; to promote the role of women as agents of change; to make their health and social needs a top priority; and to equip them with equal access to information, to technical and economic resources, and to skills, education, and opportunities. This is necessary not only for the benefit of women but for the benefit of all people and future generations.

Trends in new technologies (5,28)

Advanced technologies have wrought substantial changes in economic and social life in the past two or three decades. The introduction and dissemination of new technologies in developing countries have been fast in some cases but slow in others. Recent advances in technology have enhanced productivity and intensified communication throughout the world. Science and technology policies have become part of both the socioeconomic and political agendas in all countries. Technological change has provided hope for solving crucial economic problems and enriching people's lives, and governments have been trying to anticipate and prevent adverse and possibly enduring effects of these changes. In developed market economies innovations continued to be stimulated both by market forces and by government efforts such as funding for fundamental research and the spon-

soring of military-oriented research and development. Among the developing countries, only a few have the physical and human resources to undertake significant industrial research on their own. However, some of the largest developing countries, for example Brazil, China, India, and Mexico, have been able to catch up in certain sectors of scientific research and have a scientific and industrial infrastructure that is relatively advanced. Several of the newly industrializing economies, such as Hong Kong, the Republic of Korea and Singapore, have assimilated microelectronic-based technologies, applying them to new products and production processes.

Rapid advances in medical technology, biotechnology, equipment for diagnosis and curative procedures, transplants of a more complex nature, and new types and applications of computer-designed drugs and other new materials have greatly expanded the capabilities of modern medicine. The complicated and costly technologies involved in such research and development tend to restrict it to countries with well-developed scientific resources. However, the more widespread application of this research will eventually have a major impact on health and medical services in all countries. Chapter 4, dealing with health resources, elaborates on further advances in and applications of medical and health technologies.

In the field of education, several pilot projects related to computer use in education in developing countries have demonstrated both benefits and difficulties. The latter included lack of qualified human resources, and inadequate adaptation of software to the country's cultural environment. In developing countries the gradual introduction of microcomputers led to an increase in the demand for personnel who could work with computers in schools. But even in Brazil, which was one of the pioneers in the developing world in adopting a national policy on informatics and whose producers were supplying a growing share of this market for computer hardware, there were difficulties in the introduction of computers in teacher-training courses, despite their prior introduction in high schools.

Technological advances made possible the discovery and commercial use of a variety of new materials and have reduced the production costs of many conventional materials. At the same time, there was also a constant search for new uses for both old materials and new. Among the important groups of new materials were metals and alloys with superior strength and resistance to corrosion, and structural ceramics with superior resistance to heat, wear, and corrosion, which made them potentially important substitutes for metals. Recent discoveries of new types of superconducting materials might also eventually revolutionize electronics, power transmission, and transport.

The production of high-yielding crops based on an expanded use of irrigation and improved fertilizers, pesticides, and herbicides – the so-called "green revolution" – has been extremely beneficial in increasing supplies of food and other crops. It has considerably changed food availability in many countries, particularly in the 1980s in the Asian subcontinent and China. As biotechnology promises to transform agriculture and society at large even more dramatically, concerns are being voiced about the ecological and ethical implications of agricultural biotechnology, including the unpredictable effects of altered life forms. Among the developing countries, China has established research facilities dealing with agrobiological genetics and India has committed itself to developing large-scale programmes for creating a biotechnology industry. Biotechnology programmes have also been launched in Argentina, Brazil, Cuba, Mongolia, the Philippines, the Republic of Korea, and Thailand.

Rapid advances in technology during the past two or three decades, while distinctly enlarging production frontiers and broadening choice, have raised several questions of major importance in economic and social policy. Innovations in technology tend to make existing technology obsolete and call for new investment and new skills. In developing countries, the absorption of new technologies has been varied. In some countries, advanced technology has permeated a wide array of activities while in other countries it remains confined to a few activities, usually concentrated in large urban centres. In the more affluent societies, concern about the smooth absorption of advanced technology has been at the forefront of public discussions. Efforts towards improvements in the education system or educational reforms in recent decades to a large extent emerge from the perceived need to change the content and methods of instruction to take full advantage of new technologies. The development of new technologies holds promise for an improved quality of life worldwide. But related environmental, ethical, trade and social issues must be carefully monitored to avoid negative effects. Government policy and producer responses to the demand for new skills, new equipment, and new institutional forms will largely determine the pace of technological progress. Yet individual and social attitudes to the development and use of new technologies will continue to influence that pace. Technology has never been socially neutral. In the "global village" that is being created, the fear of cultural dominance has taken on a new dimension: the threat of the disappearance of cultural and social diversity among nations.

Intersectoral cooperation

The relationship between health status and socioeconomic development has been amply demonstrated. In developed countries, the communicable diseases that were once the principal causes of mortality were controlled by improvements in living conditions, nutritional status, sanitation, and health behaviour, and this was done before major discoveries were made regarding their cure and treatment. In the low-income countries, health development became part of the national economic strategy, which sought to provide the poor with access to resources and economic opportunities, raise educational levels, ensure the availability and distribution of food, improve the status of women, and provide the basic infrastructure of transport and other public amenities.

While the primary responsibility for achieving health goals is with the health sector and its agencies, a share of the responsibility devolves on other sectors. The past decade has seen the evolution of a wide variety of mechanisms for promoting intersectoral action. However, the conventional chain of command and organizational structure of ministries and government offices are strongly protective of departmental boundaries and therefore have built-in biases against intersectoral coordination and are not naturally responsive to objectives outside their sphere of authority. Therefore these mechanisms for the most part did not foster the dialogue on common issues, or identify the joint action required, or formulate common goals.

There are many other reasons why intersectoral health strategies have not advanced. Firstly, health planning has remained a more or less self-contained exercise within the health sector, carried out principally by health professionals in relative isolation from other development processes. This isolation is reinforced by the tendency of most sectors to perceive health as comprised mainly of medical services and their output. Secondly, there is confusion created by the use of the term "health" to mean health status, health services, and even sometimes the health sector itself. Yet each of these is clearly quite different. Whereas health services are primarily the responsibility of the health sector, health status is not. Health status is the outcome of several developmental and behavioural activities. In this context it becomes the shared responsibility of development sectors rather than the concern of the health sector alone.

The analysis and evaluation of development policies tend not to examine health outcomes.

An example of this is government pesticide subsidies, which are intended to increase agricultural productivity but which are not examined for their health impact. This is despite the fact that various consequences of increased pesticide use are well documented; they include accidental poisoning, effects on the resistance to pesticides of disease vectors, and overreliance on chemical pest control strategies when other measures might be applied more safely and at lower cost.

Research on health problems in developing countries tends not to address the role of development policies as an underlying cause of ill-health. In the 1980s the debt crisis and subsequent adjustment programmes led many organizations and individuals to criticize adjustment policies for their negative impacts on the health and nutrition of poor populations in developing countries. However, in other areas, such as industry, policy analyses have focused on epidemiological studies of occupational diseases and accidents, and have rarely explored the underlying causes of the rapid increases in ill-health. Researchers have tended to emphasize the need for health policy interventions rather than to examine the overall strategies in industrial development for their health consequences.

Even when knowledge exists on the health impacts of development policies, many obstacles may block the effective implementation of policy changes to improve health. There may, for example, be uncertainty about the health impacts of policy measures, or there may be a conflict between the economic and political interests supporting certain national goals and the policies needed to reduce pollution, accidents, and other health risks to workers or communities.

References

1. Renner, M. Enhancing global security. In: *State of the world, 1989.* New York, Norton, 1990.
2. *Development cooperation – 1990 report.* Paris, Organization for Economic Co-operation and Development, 1990.

3. *Asia 1991 yearbook.* Hong Kong, Far Eastern Economic Review, 1991.

4. *The challenge to the South. Report of the South Commission.* New York, Oxford University Press, 1990.

5. *Global outlook 2000 – an economic, social and environmental perspective.* New York, United Nations, 1990.

6. *World economic survey.* New York, United Nations, 1991.

7. *Trade and development report 1991.* New York, United Nations Commission for Trade and Development, 1991.

8. *The least developed countries – 1990 report.* New York, United Nations Commission for Trade and Development, 1991.

9. *Report of the Committee for Development Planning on its twenty-seventh session, 22–26 April 1991.* New York, United Nations, 1991 (document E/1991/32).

10. *World development report 1990.* Washington, DC, World Bank, 1990.

11. *The social dimensions of adjustment – a policy agenda.* Draft paper by United Nations Development Programme/African Development Bank/World Bank, November 1989 (document RAF/86/037/A/01/42).

12. *Official records of the General Assembly.* Forty-fifth session, United Nations, 11 October 1990 [supplement No. 41(A/45/41)].

13. *Planning for balanced economic and social development: six country case studies.* New York, United Nations, 1964; *Unified socioeconomic development and planning: some new horizons.* New York, United Nations, 1971 (International social development review No. 3); McGranahan, D.V. et al. *Contents and measurement of socioeconomic development.* New York, Praeger, 1972; *Report on a unified approach to development and planning.* New York, United Nations, 1974 (document E/CN.5/519, 5 December 1974); *Application by governments of a unified approach to development analysis and planning.* Report of the Secretary-General. New York, United Nations, 1976 (document E/CN.540, 22 September 1976); *World development report 1982.* Washington, DC, World Bank, 1982.

14. *World development report 1991.* Washington, DC, World Bank, 1991.

15. *Investing in the future – setting educational priorities in the developing world.* Paris, Pergamon Press, 1990.

16. Drewnowski, J. & Subramanian, M. Social aims in development plans. In: *Studies in the methodology of social planning.* Geneva, United Nations Research Institute for Social Development, 1970 (report No. 70.5).

17. *World population prospects 1990.* New York, United Nations, 1991.

18. *World urbanization prospects 1990.* New York, United Nations, 1991.

19. *The state of the world environment.* Nairobi, United Nations Environment Programme, 1987.

20. *World population monitoring 1991.* United Nations, 14 January 1991 (draft document ESA/P/WP.114).

21. *Food outlook, No. 1–2.* Rome, Food and Agriculture Organization, 1991.

22. Barraclough, S. *The end to hunger? The social origins of food strategies.* ZED Books, 1991.

23. *Production yearbook 1989.* Rome, Food and Agriculture Organization, 1990.

24. *Statistical yearbook 1990.* Paris, United Nations Educational, Scientific and Cultural Organization, 1990.

25. *Economically active population: estimates and projections, 1950–2025.* Geneva, International Labour Organisation, 1986.

26. *Safety and health of migrant workers – an international symposium.* Geneva, International Labour Organisation, 1979.

27. Birks, J.S. & Sinclair, C.A. *Manpower and population evolution in the GCC and the Libyan Arab Jamahiriya.* Geneva, World Employment Programme Research, 1989 (working paper).

28. *1989 report on the world social situation.* New York, United Nations, 1989.

CHAPTER 2

Development of health systems

Health for all and the development of health systems

The concept of primary health care, as outlined in the report of a joint WHO/UNICEF conference in Alma-Ata, USSR, in 1978, was a breakthrough towards a worldwide movement to reduce the gap between "haves" and "have-nots", popularly known as Health for All by the Year 2000 (HFA 2000).

The Minister of Health of Trinidad and Tobago, President of the World Health Assembly in 1979, expressed his hope and voiced his pride at taking part in "laying the foundations of a truly worldwide philosophy of justice in health with the accompanying political will to act". Countries were fully aware of the weight of their decision: as one delegate said, "The path to health for all will be extraordinarily steep and difficult … [but] … we have had the judgement and genius, the goodwill and good sense to set our concern about the health of humanity and our commitment to improve health everywhere on earth above narrow political considerations".

Based on the global strategy for health for all launched in 1981, countries were invited to review their health systems with the aim of reshaping them as necessary in conformity with the agreed essential characteristics of the health system (*1*).

For the development of a health system conforming to a set of basic principles (see box), most Member States began to prepare first their own national policies, strategies, and plans of

---

Basic principles for the development of health systems (1)

- The system should encompass the entire population on the basis of equality and reciprocity.

- The system should include components from the health sector and from other sectors whose interrelated actions contribute to health.

- Primary health care should consist of at least the essential elements enunciated in the Declaration of Alma-Ata.

- The other elements of the health system should support the first contact level of primary health care to permit it to provide these essential elements on a continuing basis.

- At intermediate levels, more complex problems should be dealt with, more skilled and specialized care as well as logistic support should be provided, and more highly trained staff should provide continuing training to primary health care workers – as well as guidance to communities and community health workers on practical problems arising in connection with all aspects of primary health care.

- The central level should coordinate all parts of the system and provide planning and management expertise in aspects that are common to all institutions in the country.

action, and then regional and global strategies for attaining an acceptable level of health for all by the year 2000. Some countries prepared national strategies after regional (and global) strategies had been formulated.

Equity in health, defined as "the universal coverage of the population, with care provided according to need" (2), was recognized as being an important objective in the achievement of health for all in order to reduce the gaps between countries and between different groups within countries.

Countries have been approaching their formidable task in a variety of ways best suited to their own context such as providing the full range of services required, starting with those in greatest need and progressively reaching the whole population, or providing limited services to the total population from the beginning and progressively extending the range of services. In all cases it was found that a sound health system infrastructure is necessary to sustain the implementation of activities.

A "midpoint" review of progress was carried out at Riga, USSR, in 1988 (2). It became clear that there was no common understanding of the meaning of health for all through primary health care. But one way or another, all countries have tried to translate the rhetoric of health for all into reality at all levels – country, regional, and global. All sectors of activity have become aware of their responsibility for health, and the public has become increasingly well informed about healthy behaviour. In villages, towns, and districts, people are waking up to the fact that they can contribute to their own health development.

Now, 15 years after Alma-Ata, all countries accept that primary health care (see box) is the basic tool needed to achieve health for all.

Political commitment to achieving health for all through primary health care is only a first step. It must be followed by implementation of the strategy, cutting across economic, political, and other boundaries.

Primary health care (3)

Primary health care is essential health care based on practical, scientifically sound and socially acceptable methods and technology made universally accessible to individuals and families in the community through their full participation and at a cost that the community and country can afford ... It forms an integral part both of the country's health system, of which it is the central function and main focus, and of the overall social and economic development of the community.

Primary health care ... includes at least:

- education concerning prevailing health problems and the methods of preventing and controlling them;
- promotion of food supply and proper nutrition;
- an adequate supply of safe water and basic sanitation;
- maternal and child health care, including family planning;
- immunization against the major infectious diseases;
- prevention and control of locally endemic diseases;
- appropriate treatment of common diseases and injuries;
- provision of essential drugs.

The time has come to assess progress in implementing what appears to be a near-Utopian philosophy, especially in the current socioeconomic context where one step forward seems often to be followed by two steps back. It is to be hoped that countries will soldier on with courage towards the goal of health for all, however distant it may seem. Had they considered only the constraints and not the opportunities, they would never have defined the policies they did or adopted such ambitious goals.

How the strategy for health for all is being implemented

The global strategy for health for all was formulated in 1981 (*1*). Since then, Member States have made concerted efforts to implement it

---

Global targets (1)

1. All people in every country will have ready access at least to essential health care and to first-level referral facilities.

2. All people will be actively involved in caring for themselves and their families as far as they can and in community action for health.

3. Communities throughout the world will share with governments responsibility for the health care of their members.

4. All governments will assume overall responsibility for the health of their people.

5. Safe drinking-water and sanitation will be available to all people.

6. All people will be adequately nourished.

7. All children will be immunized against the major infectious diseases of childhood.

8. Communicable diseases in the developing countries will be of no greater public health significance in the year 2000 than they are in developed countries in the year 1980.

9. All possible ways will be applied to prevent and control noncommunicable diseases and promote mental health through influencing life styles and controlling the physical and psychosocial environment.

10. Essential drugs will be available to all.

---

through country health systems based on their own national health policies and strategies. It provided global targets to be considered by Member States, taking into account their own socioeconomic and health situations and bearing in mind that all countries are aiming at the same targets for the year 2000.

In order to achieve these global targets, health plans should be developed to enable the range of health promotion, disease prevention, curative, and rehabilitative services to become available to all. The aim of a health system (see box below) is health development – the process of continuous, progressive improvement of the health status of populations (*4*).

A health system (1)

A health system consists of interrelated components that contribute to health in homes, educational institutions, workplaces, public places, and communities, as well as in the physical and psychosocial environment and the health and related sectors, like agriculture, education, environment, etc. A health system is usually organized at various levels, starting at the most peripheral level, also known as the community level or the primary level of health care, and proceeding through the intermediate (district, regional, or provincial) level to the central level. At the same time it includes individuals and families taking an active interest and participating in solving their own health problems, thus becoming full members of the health team. The intermediate and central levels deal with those elements of the health system for which they are given responsibility by the country's administrative organization, and they also provide progressively more complex and more specialized care and support.

One of the main tasks for countries in the last decade has been to develop a health system which is country, situation, and problem specific and which would, in the most efficient and effective way, try to solve priority health problems and contribute to improving health status.

In an effort to develop and build up their health systems based on primary health care, countries have reviewed existing systems with the aim of reorganizing them to tackle inequities in health by involving people within the community, supported by the health services and have tried to cover the whole population.

During the first evaluation of the strategy for health for all, in 1985, the main emphasis was on processes and on their compatibility with the principles of health for all, with some reflections on their adequacy for achieving that goal. This second evaluation aims at assessing the practical implementation of these strategies – to discover, in short, what has been achieved and, if something has not been achieved, why it has not. This should enable Member States and WHO to suggest measures and actions for more appropriate and effective implementation of the strategy.

Of the 12 global indicators to be used in evaluating the strategy, the three dealing with

the implementation of policies and strategies and the health system are used to evaluate the development of health systems (see box).

Health policies and strategies

The major focus of this section is on the ways in which policies and strategies have been implemented with regard to: (1) endorsement of health-for-all policy, (2) equity in health, (3) allocation and distribution of resources for primary health care, and (4) leadership development.

There have been some difficulties in analysing country information. For example, some countries have a national policy which is actually entitled "Health for All", others have national health policies which clearly make specific reference to it, and yet others did not specifically refer to health for all in their reports though they clearly reflected its principles in their health policies.

Using the global policy and strategy as a guide, most countries have formulated national health policies and are committed to translating them into action through country development plans.

Endorsement of health-for-all policy

The policy continues to receive endorsement at the highest level – in the United Nations, at all meetings of WHO governing bodies, and in national parliaments and legislatures. In the 151 country reports so far reviewed, continuous endorsement is mentioned in 110, no endorsement in four, and "not known/no information" in 37 (see Annex table: global indicator 1).

In some countries, health-for-all policy has been endorsed since 1983 (Austria, India). In some others, political leaders frequently make statements in support of it (Cuba, Iran), while in others its policy and strategy are endorsed and accepted by parliaments or governments (Norway, Sierra Leone). Although 28 countries did not give specific information in their reports, it

---

> **Global indicators dealing with health systems**
>
> No. 1 The number of countries in which health for all is continuing to receive endorsement at the highest level.
>
> No. 2 The number of countries in which mechanisms for involving people in the implementation of strategies are fully functioning or are being further developed.
>
> No. 5 The number of countries in which resources for primary health care are becoming more equitably distributed.

could be assumed that they are committed to health for all by their endorsement of the Declaration of Alma-Ata and subsequent WHA resolutions, approved by their delegations or through their Regional Committees or in special initiatives such as Bamako (1987), where endorsement was reconfirmed collectively by countries in Africa.[1]

In some countries, such as Bangladesh, health for all by the year 2000 through primary health care has been accepted as a national goal but a formal health policy document has yet to be issued. In Bhutan, the health-for-all policy document is in preparation. Some countries reported no official endorsement. Qatar said it did not need to revise its strategies in view of its small land area and population.

Most countries reported that a better climate for the implementation of national health policies and strategies had been created by increased awareness and better understanding of primary health care.

Although the majority of countries have accepted that health development is important for overall socioeconomic development, some reported resistance to health-for-all policies by some sectors. For example, Zimbabwe notes that some economists and development planners are increasingly voicing the opinion that health is not a productive sector and that national resources should be devoted to productive sectors of the economy. In some countries, resistance to health for all and primary health care comes from within the health sector – mostly from the clinically oriented medical profession.

Health policy development in some countries has been closely linked to analysis and evaluation of the health situation, and new health policies and plans have been adopted on

this basis (as in Oman in 1989 and Pakistan in 1990), or on the basis of extensive health reports (as in France). Member States in south-east Asia have taken effective steps to integrate the policies and strategies adopted in the health sector into overall national development policies. In the Far East and the Pacific, health for all through primary health care is the basis for national health development in all countries and areas.

When moving from policy and strategy to implementation, a number of countries have been adversely affected by economic recession or war, which has made it difficult to sustain existing programmes, and some of them have already modified their strategies to cope with emerging problems.

In some developing and least developed countries – where available resources are very limited – implementation is concentrated on developing the relatively weak infrastructure, improving coverage, supporting decentralization, and integrating programmes, especially at district and peripheral level.

Experience over many years from some developing countries (Costa Rica and Kerala State in India) has shown that with political will and good management the implementation of appropriate strategies, emphasizing education, the involvement of the people, and intersectoral collaboration, can lead to a rapid improvement in health status, especially among vulnerable groups, in spite of limited resources.

In developed and in some developing countries, health-for-all policies are used to further promote health in areas such as environment, life style, mental health, and disabilities. In the United States, a new policy "Healthy people 2000" was launched in 1990, based on experience in the implementation of strategies and programmes in the 1980s.

Good progress in implementation of national strategies was reported by most European countries, although explicitly formulated health-for-all strategies do not always exist.

---

1. The Bamako initiative, launched in 1987 in collaboration with WHO and UNICEF, aimed at mobilizing funds to improve maternal and child care as part of primary health care in Africa, particularly through the release of funds from recovering the cost of essential drugs as well as other cost-effective mechanisms.

This is the case in Denmark, but it is not considered an obstacle to establishing mechanisms and activities in line with health for all.

Some countries have experienced considerable political, social, and economic changes recently, especially in eastern Europe. Although national health strategies and plans have been revised and adjusted in keeping with new political, social, economic, and managerial realities, progress in implementation has been slowed down.

In order to cope with new and important emerging priority problems, many countries have developed policies for specific sectors such as food, nutrition, and the environment, with emphasis on implementation of these policies. This can be considered as a bridge for intersectoral collaboration, which will allow different advisory and coordinating mechanisms to be established.

Overall, commitment to and endorsement of health for all are considered by almost all Member States to be important steps towards implementing the strategy, although success in implementation is less evident, as indicated in the following sections.

Equity in health

Differences between the "haves" and "have-nots" in health status and in access to food, clean water, and health services, have always existed both between and within countries. In the Declaration of Alma-Ata inequities in the health status of the people were identified as a common concern of all countries (see box).

The Thirty-ninth World Health Assembly (1986), recalling that existing inequalities in health are unacceptable, called on Member States "to include in their health-for-all strategy specific equity-oriented targets expressed in terms of improved health among disadvantaged groups such as women, the rural poor, the inhabitants of urban slums, and the people engaged in hazardous occupations" and also urged Member States "to maintain high-level

> **From the Declaration of Alma-Ata (3)**
>
> The existing gross inequality in the health status of the people particularly between developed and developing countries as well as within countries is politically, socially and economically unacceptable and is, therefore, of common concern to all countries.

political commitment to social equity" (resolutions WHA39.22 and WHA39.7).

The Forty-second World Health Assembly (1989) noted the progress made, but recognized the need to accelerate implementation of the strategy and urged Member States "to maintain the political commitment to reduce the inequities among the different population groups" (resolution WHA42.2).

As a result of increasing awareness of and concern for the issue of equity, countries intensified their action to improve the existing situation. Government responsibility and measures taken for reducing existing inequities in health vary from country to country. Some countries are trying to develop policies and strategies dealing with disadvantaged groups, while others have set targets to decrease the inequities. All countries consider involvement of the people in their communities, involvement of nongovernmental organizations and other agencies, and also collaboration with other sectors to be important prerequisites for decreasing inequities in health.

Some countries have started to develop programmes intended to reduce inequities, based on better information, to enable them to take active measures (including legislation) or to monitor progress.

In many developing and least developed countries, efforts are being made to improve the health situation of the rural population, urban slum dwellers, and some vulnerable groups and to identify groups for special support such as migrants, nomads, and those living in geo-graphically remote areas.

China, in spite of great advances, reports an imbalance between regions. Rural health services are identified as a priority, but since financial management is decentralized, there can be discrepancies between regions owing to their economic status, so that unbalanced development of health services may be aggravated. "The uneven socioeconomic development in different areas has led to a serious variation in health conditions. The problems of unavailability of medical services and drugs in a few areas have not been radically solved. There is a big gap in the entitlement of medical care between urban and rural inhabitants. The distribution of health resources is extremely uneven". Mongolia reports difficulties in reaching the semi-nomads (cattle breeders) who represent nearly half the population as they move from one place to another throughout the year and always live at some distance from district or subdistrict centres.

In some countries, a health policy promoting equitable distribution of resources has been developed, but because of geographical inaccessibility or war it is difficult to implement. In other countries, the priority area for the ministry of health is the reduction in inequity, but the main problem resides in the method of resource allocation. In many countries, rich and poor, owing to political changes and growth in unemployment, a further deterioration in the health status of the elderly, the unemployed, and the disabled or the lower socioeconomic groups has been noticed.

The United States, noting that 30–37 million citizens have no health insurance, reports that, for the 1990s, the country's health agencies are strongly committed to narrowing the gap between the total population and "population groups at special risk", such as people with low incomes, people who are members of some racial/ethnic minority group, and people with disabilities.

European countries, recognizing "a glaring inequity in health", collectively agreed in 1984 to set the following target: "by the year 2000, to reduce actual differences in health status between countries and between groups within countries by at least 25%, by improving the level of health of disadvantaged nations and groups".

These countries have mentioned difficulties in measuring equity, and only during recent years has more attention been paid to empirical data. Studies focused on equity are reported from several countries. Excess ill-health among ethnic minorities and immigrants are mentioned by Israel, Switzerland, and the United Kingdom. Sweden considers equity in health to be an overriding priority in view of increasing inequity in the 1980s. There is a need to improve the working environment to help reduce differences between occupational groups. The Netherlands has established a programme committee on socioeconomic differences in health, and data on any health differentials that have been found are made available to the municipalities, who then decide on the measures required. Norway also has developed a special project aimed at reducing inequities.

Australia reports that a major challenge is to help more effectively groups that are significantly disadvantaged (Aborigines, Torres Strait islanders), groups with the lowest health status, and low socioeconomic groups, including recent migrants.

Differences in levels of health between and within countries still remain and are a cause of concern for governments in both developing and developed countries. Few countries have adequate data on the health of some groups such as the underprivileged, gaps are not narrowing or are even widening, and, even in countries where targets for reduction of the differences in health status exist, these improvements may be difficult to achieve.

Bearing in mind that no single measure of equity exists at present and that there may be different patterns in different countries, it is evident that the question of equity needs not only special attention from national authorities but also international solidarity and support. Clearly, too, there is a need to develop methods and measures for improvement that are appropriate, relevant, selective, and even specific to particular countries and areas.

Allocation and distribution of resources for primary health care

Political commitment to health for all is reflected by trends in the allocation and distribution of resources. Reports from 32 countries stated that resources are more equitably distributed towards primary health care. In 108 reports, however, information on resource allocation for primary health care was not provided, and in 11 reports answers were negative (see Annex table: global indicator 5).

Even among the countries that did not make specific statements about resources, some have indicated indirectly that there is a tendency for more equitable distribution of resources for primary health care. The Bahamas, for example, reported increased allocation to community health services, and Bolivia indicated that health facilities had been established in rural areas. On the other hand Ethiopia reports that there has been no significant change in distribution of resources towards the rural areas of the country. Reasons given by countries that reported negatively about equitable distribution for primary health care included the statement that efforts are still under way and that the vast majority of resources for such care come from external sources.

Some developing and least developed countries reported that resources for primary health care are better distributed with respect to the rural population and that more have been allocated to preventive measures (Malawi), or that resources have been distributed evenly to all provinces based on agreed criteria (Indonesia).

Some countries have increased their share of resources to underprivileged population groups, particularly urban slum dwellers, nomads, and inhabitants of sparsely-populated remote areas. For example, Saudi Arabia has expressed concern about nomads and is carrying out research on how to extend services to them, while Egypt encourages visits by health care staff to sensitive population groups and Oman has mobile teams ("flying squads") to reach isolated localities.

A majority of developed countries have indicated that resources for primary health care are distributed evenly to all regions or provinces and also that resources are decentralized, as for example in Finland, where attention has been paid to a specific strategy for the elderly and disabled, equity between regions has been further emphasized, and resources have been reallocated to certain areas on the basis of needs.

In spite of general agreement that available resources should be more equitably distributed for primary health care, reallocation of these resources has not been easy. Some constraints mentioned by countries are: (1) lack of realistic resource planning, (2) lack of criteria for more even distribution, (3) lack of motivation of health personnel to work at the peripheral level, and (4) insufficient resources to permit the necessary redistribution.

Leadership development

Attainment of the goal of health for all will depend on the existence of a critical group of people who can conceive and implement national strategies.

Colloquia and dialogues have brought together groups of individuals (policy- and decision-makers, senior and middle-level health administrators, community leaders, and heads of educational institutions and training programmes) to engage them in dialogues on national health-for-all issues as they apply to their own situations.

Countries in south-east Asia have been extremely active. For example, a number of national workshops on leadership training within the health sector have been held in Bangladesh,

Regional initiatives

Each of the WHO Regions has evolved a different focus and framework for leadership development activities, depending on socioeconomic, political, and global factors.

The **African Region** organized an informal consultation with members of the African Advisory Committee for Health Development to discuss a strategy for pursuing leadership development. Most activities have stressed the intersectoral nature of health and the need to strengthen leadership at district level. This has been done by emphasizing management training, and the Regional Office has funded a number of seminars and workshops both at country and intercountry level.

The **Region of the Americas** has been promoting leadership development through the Research Training Programme in International Health and advanced training for policy-makers in international health. Emphasis has been put on examining the political process, issues of resource allocation in the light of current economic constraints and debt-restructuring, and sensitizing politicians and policy-makers from health and other key sectors to the issues at hand. Further, the Organization has held informal consultations on leadership development in educational institutions with representatives of the Latin American and United States Associations of Schools of Public Health, in order to explore the possibilities of organizing international and regional courses.

The **South-East Asia Region** has established an ad hoc working group on leadership development, which prepared a regional plan emphasizing training activities at all levels in the health sector. A number of regional conferences, intercountry workshops, and national seminars have been supported with the aim of sensitizing policy-makers and training a core group of faciliators in leadership development.

In the **European Region**, the Regional Office has used health-for-all policy reviews in several countries as opportunities for active dialogue with national policy-makers. In addition, health policy dialogues for parliamentarians and senior policy-makers have been organized in order to discuss the kinds of policy changes needed to reach agreed health targets. Emphasis has also been placed on leadership as a means of strengthening intersectoral action for health development.

In the **Eastern Mediterranean Region**, the Regional Committee endorsed a recommendation that 10% of the fellowship allocations be used for health leadership development. A nine-month residency programme in health leadership development is planned per biennium. Concurrently, this Region has organized intercountry workshops on leadership development in an effort to build up core groups of facilitators at national level.

The **Western Pacific Region** focuses on training young professionals in international health, and has also initiated a regional health management development network in the South Pacific with emphasis on developing human resources and improving their leadership capacities.

while in Bhutan, annual workshops of senior district health officers (*dzongdas*), medical officers, and district health officers have been held, as well as workshops for intermediate-level health staff and community leaders, training and refresher courses for health staff and volunteer workers, and participation of communities in planning and development of rural areas.

India, Myanmar, and Nepal have accelerated their training activities. Seminars for parliamentarians and regional and district administrative and political personnel have been organized in Sri Lanka. In Thailand, one of the most successful activities at national level has been the training of 400 leaders in a metropolitan Bangkok slum improvement project.

A national coordinating mechanism has been established by the Ministry of Health of Indonesia to coordinate the planning, implementation, and evaluation of an HFA leadership development programme at national level.

In the Middle East, activities in Afghanistan, Iran, Jordan, Saudi Arabia, and Yemen have focused on advocacy at policy-making levels, and training in leadership skills for middle-level and community-level health personnel.

In China, a programme of health-for-all leadership development was undertaken in three provinces where special emphasis was placed on promoting primary health care to a wide intersectoral audience, and in 1988, the Ministry of Public Health, with WHO collaboration, sponsored a high-level seminar for provincial leaders throughout the country.

In all probability, very few of the changes in national policy that have resulted in implementation of primary health care have taken place without the involvement of senior government and nongovernment officials in intercountry visits and dialogues of the types described here. Another direct result of the regional or intercountry meetings has been the organization of many different activities at country level, seeking to educate and influence health-related personnel at all levels towards health-for-all values and principles.

Organization of health systems based on primary health care

Achieving the goal of health for all by the year 2000 requires concerted efforts from countries to organize their health systems based on primary health care. The past decade has seen both solid progress and serious setbacks. Some countries maintain a priority commitment to such care and can demonstrate success in improving the accessibility and quality of health care. In others, falling living standards, massive indebtedness, and ecological decline have had a negative impact on both health services and health status.

In spite of improvements, there is still a big gap in many countries between the acceptance of the principles of primary health care and their implementation in the development of policies, financing, organization, management, and the delivery of programmes.

Ingredients of success in developing health systems

Looking back over the past 5 years, the successful development of health systems based on primary health care appears to be due to the following factors:

- government, political, social and financial commitment;
- strong management capabilities for implementation;
- well-oriented, trained, and committed health personnel;
- decentralization to district/local level;
- community involvement in local decisions;
- sustained financing;
- the widespread deployment of affordable life-saving technologies.

Five global changes in the second half of the 1980s have had a direct impact on health system development. Economically, there has been a marked decline in developing countries. Significant demographic changes include rapid urbanization and particularly the growth of peri-urban areas and a global increase in the number of people aged 65 and over. Environmental degradation poses an increasing threat to health in many parts of the world. People have become much more aware of health, and their demands for and expectations of quality services and care have likewise increased. Also, people outside the formal health sector are becoming actively involved in decisions about and action for their health, as evidenced, for example, by the large number of nongovernmental organizations now involved in health care.

The majority of countries are trying to further reorient their health systems towards primary health care. Its principles are generally well understood and accepted, particularly by paramedical staff, but some curative-oriented medical staff at the highest level still promote second- and third-level care to the detriment of first-level care. In a number of countries, however, first-level care is a priority in national health system plans, and quality of care is stressed.

Many countries, including developing countries, have indicated the need to use resources more efficiently and to improve access to and the quality of health care. Quality of services is an important aspect of appropriate care, and quality assurance can now be found on the political agenda in some countries (e.g., Belgium, Indonesia, Israel, Italy, Malaysia). A number of specific approaches are fairly widely used, such as quality control in pathology laboratories, consensus reports,[1] and the collection of a minimum set of data on patients. Yet, although quality of care implies the use of appropriate health technologies, the systematic assessment of technologies (especially low-cost) remains rare.

Most countries in the Far East and the Pacific have emphasized in their reports that primary health care consists of more than the provision of various medical services and that all its eight elements must be available at community level. Steps are being taken towards decentralization, integration, and the improvement of district health systems and of the service to rural areas. Some countries report successful integration of modern and traditional medicine.

An increasing number of countries are adopting policies of decentralization aimed at improving the use of available resources for the implementation of primary health care.

In some countries, particular attention is being given to the decentralization of authority and responsibility to the district level, and different approaches have been tried in developing countries. For example, technical and managerial training to improve institutional performance has been the focus in Guinea-Bissau, Lao People's Democratic Republic, and Nigeria. In Lesotho and Zambia attention is directed to health systems research for developing improved methods and procedures to ensure that the implementation of programmes will be responsive to local needs. The strengthening of information support relevant to local needs, including related methodological tools, has been stressed in Ethiopia, Papua New Guinea, and the Philippines.

In a number of other countries there has been almost no delegation of effective power and authority to the local level, or such delegation has been only nominal, without sufficient resources or technical support from central or local levels.

Most countries expressed the conviction that district health systems are important for the organization and provision of primary health care as an integral part of the national health system and are a vital element in fostering development.

1. In the United States, for instance, the Consensus Development Conference, a key element of the consensus development programme, provides a public forum for the lay and medical community to assess new or existing technologies through an open meeting lasting two or three days.

The district is considered to be the key location in most health systems to test and consolidate primary health care, and to be a valuable bridge between the first and the other levels of care of the health system. There is considerable scope for improving management at the district level of the health system, thereby helping local health workers to perform more effectively even in the difficult circumstances they often face. The district health system is already being strengthened with various degrees of success in many countries, including Ghana, Namibia, and the Syrian Arab Republic.

In the majority of least developed countries, health system infrastructures are by and large not fully developed, and management is generally weak. Support from external resources has often been used to strengthen health system infrastructure and management, including health information systems.

In other countries, health care facilities have been broadened, with special emphasis on the rural areas, to ensure that facilities providing minimum essential health care are within easy reach. Problems with referral to a higher level are commonly reported, although well-developed referral systems have often been established to support health centres at the periphery.

In many countries curative services still predominate, to the detriment of promotive and preventive health activities. Restructuring of the health care system and decentralization of responsibility and authority to the districts have enabled some countries to start working towards integration (e.g., Nepal).

While countries are recognizing the need for increased hospital support, particularly at the first-referral level, hospitals are generally managed separately and are not yet fully integrated with other health services. The integration of health care is discussed in more detail in chapter 3.

In developed countries there is a growing awareness of the importance of efficiency, equity, and quality of care. The role of central government is shifting towards policy and strategy, while in many countries local government structures provide a wide range of services often substantially financed by local funds. Internal market mechanisms and competition are seen as additional resources for improving the performance of health services.

The need to emphasize that health and social services are resources and investments, not unproductive sectors, was mentioned in some country and regional reports. For this fact to be fully accepted and acted upon by political decision-makers, it is necessary to disseminate appropriate information and to construct mechanisms to ensure that this position is continually emphasized, regardless of the direction of reforms.

The health care reforms (including insurance and financing) now under way in Europe provide an important challenge for health for all in the 1990s. They should help:

(1) to advocate and inject into the present health care debate health-for-all principles and experience, placing the citizen in various roles and settings in the centre of such a debate (*choice, equity, participation*);

(2) to provide a clear and practical primary health care framework for new developments in health care financing; and

(3) to underline the importance of the appropriate use of financial and technological resources in increasing the efficiency of the health care system.

Some major programmes based on the primary health care approach have proved successful. In general, however, disparities and inequalities in availability of national health services have remained high and have even increased in some cases. This is partly due to the fact that an intensified effort in one programme has been accompanied by a decrease in another. The main reason for the disparities is that unnecessary, costly, and sophisticated health services are provided to some population groups, leaving fewer resources for the rest of the population.

Experience shows that progress from a vertical to an integrated approach is slow, although some improvements in coverage have been achieved by programmes following a vertical approach. Such a move is best planned from the beginning and should not be left to be considered as an afterthought.

Several Latin American countries report that there is no health system as such, but a multitude of agencies providing health care, with problems of integration and coordination, leading to increased cost and lowered efficiency.

Other constraints on the reorganization of the health system based on primary health care are the influence of pressure groups that advocate "glamorous" expensive second- and third-level care, particularly when they get the support of a sector of the medical profession trained in the strictly curative approach. These vested interests impede the implementation of primary health care.

Another group of problems have a common root, namely national economic difficulties. They are: (1) the slow expansion of services to underserved areas; (2) lack of trained and motivated staff; (3) lack of supervision; and (4) lack of transport or fuel for the referral of patients. In some Middle East countries there is also a cultural problem – the demand that service should be offered on request to anyone at an institution and at any level of care. Lastly, in a few cases, health development projects are tied to international agencies that would prefer to maintain a "vertical" structure in order to retain central control of project activities.

Managerial process

The managerial style practised in any socioeconomic sector is determined by the overall political and cultural environment in which development takes place. There is, however, general agreement on the content and different phases of the managerial process through the decision-making hierarchy. The responsibility and authority assigned to individuals in such an organizational structure may vary among countries and even among communities within a country.

Traditionally the managerial process was more often used to satisfy administrative requirements than for the development of health systems or even health services.

With the new thrust in the strategy for achieving health for all by the year 2000, it was necessary to develop the concept of broader, but practical and integrated, processes that focused on the implementation of activities for national health development, rather than health services (5).

Since the beginning of the health-for-all movement, there has been a major shift in understanding the role of management in decision-making to ensure that resources are used efficiently and effectively for health development. There are signs of improvement in health system management, which include involving communities as well as all sectors relevant to health and ensuring reallocation of resources to health development priorities.

A number of Member States reported their concern to strengthen the managerial capacity of their health systems and further improve managerial processes. In some developed countries, permanent mechanisms to provide political and technical support as well as effective coordination within the health sector are established, while in others, in spite of improvements in managerial processes, permanent mechanisms do not yet exist. Planning, analytical, and coordinating capacities, especially at the intermediate and peripheral levels (including community), are still considered weak in many countries and need significant improvement.

A growing number of countries have realized the potential contribution of economic principles to their managerial process. Several have elaborated a strategy for cost containment, and some have devised a master plan for financing health for all. In a context of lasting economic strain, many of them are still searching for different ways of financing their health care services.

A more recent trend is to focus on improving management of district health systems using certain innovations such as active problem-solving by district teams, which are producing encouraging results, at least in the short term. Lack of trained health managers for all levels is reported by the majority of developing and least developed countries. So far, more emphasis is being placed on training for health managers at central and intermediate than at lower levels. Learning by doing and problem-solving based on health care practice in the country are slowly superseding traditional training approaches.

In many countries, continuous monitoring and evaluation constitute an integral component of the managerial process and are often carried out by the department responsible for planning in the ministries of health. Although they are recognized as important tools for the rapid, dynamic, and permanent improvement of health programme implementation, they are still not being used fully for decentralized management by the health system to match local needs and priorities with national policy guidelines and resource allocation.

In a majority of African countries there is a need to intensify efforts to strengthen management capacities at all levels of the national health system to build up appropriate managerial mechanisms for improving coordination within the health sector and among other sectors, including involvement of communities. Emphasis has been laid on the decentralization of the managerial process and monitoring of the progress of primary health care, which is gradually being introduced by all African Member States.

In many countries of the Americas, administrative reforms to rationalize health expenditure, to transfer some responsibility for health services management and financing to the private sector or to communities, are under way. Reforms aimed at the decentralization of author-

ity have accompanied the democratization process.

A number of countries in the Middle East have reviewed and tried to strengthen and reorient their health information systems, to solve management problems. Many of these countries reported a lack of staff trained in health information and mentioned that management cannot function properly without adequate information support, i.e., without a health information system capable of making available relevant, reliable information at the right time, to the right person, in a usable form, and at an affordable cost. Member States have taken initiatives to develop their information systems. Oman, for example, is on the way to having a regional health information system to support regionalization of its health system.

In south-east Asian countries, the core of management capacity has been developed at national level and it is now necessary to focus more on intermediate and local levels. Planning units have recently been reorganized in the ministries of health of some countries (e.g., Sri Lanka), while in Myanmar, the managerial process has been reoriented to cope with emerging priority problems and needs. In India and Nepal, revised health management information systems have been expanded and implemented as a centrally supported scheme. Improved information support to health management is frequently related to finances, but it also includes the epidemiological data needed to assess the country's situation and take necessary measures.

A number of countries in the Far East and the Pacific (American Samoa, Kiribati, Malaysia, Philippines, Solomon Islands, Tonga, and Vanuatu) are making efforts to improve the managerial process by strengthening the planning component. Recent developments in this area include increasing the participation of other agencies in planning, as in Tonga, and expanding the planning process to the regional and provincial levels of the system, as in the Philippines. The common feature of these countries is that the responsibility and accountability for resource utilization has been delegated outside the central level.

In some European countries (e.g., Sweden) there is a tendency to challenge existing managerial processes by shifting emphasis in health planning towards revised or new strategies, and from monitoring outputs towards evaluating outcomes (impacts). In a number of countries of this region, central control versus decentralization has long been an important political and organizational issue. There has been a widespread trend towards decentralization in health management from the centre to regions, provinces, and districts. The common feature in some of these countries is that responsibility and accountability for resource utilization has been delegated to the district level. Some countries in eastern Europe have already introduced health reforms that include managerial changes as key elements, including improvement of the health management information system.

Discrepancies are still observed however between health policy statements on the one hand and health resource allocation and activities implemented by priority programmes on the other. Despite the sincere efforts of Member States to improve and strengthen the managerial processes, especially monitoring and evaluation, various problems have been recognized as impediments to the effective management of health systems based on primary health care. The development of a satisfactory managerial process has often been hampered by the scarcity of skilled planners, but also by poor linkage between planners, implementers, and decision-makers. Lack of qualified staff trained in management (particularly at provincial and district levels) is a common problem, often aggravated by another one – the frequent change in management personnel.

Weak management at the district (or operational) level was not always improved by the creation of district management teams or similar action. Unless full responsibility and account-

ability are given to the programme managers at the delivery level, any improvement in this area may not have the desired effect.

Another important and long-standing issue is weak health information systems or lack of adequate information support (or the other extreme of excessive data collection with limited utilization and limited feedback), which is a significant obstacle to successful management. This often exists together with insufficient technical and financial resources, so that the integration of monitoring and evaluation within the managerial process is still unsatisfactory.

Community involvement

The Alma-Ata conference defined community involvement as a process whereby communities, families, and individuals assume responsibility for their own health and welfare and develop the capacity to contribute to their own and the community's development. Communities should be involved in assessing their health situation, defining the problems, planning priorities, implementing activities, and monitoring and evaluating their own programmes. To succeed in this, all involved – individuals, families, communities, and society as a whole – must develop such mechanisms, based on clearly defined objectives, mutual interest, good understanding, and collaboration, as will permit the effective implementation of agreed programme activities.

Mechanisms for community involvement should be adapted to local circumstances and needs, so there cannot be one universal model. The major approaches to community involvement in primary health care may be categorized broadly into several models. It should be emphasized that any categorization has limitations and that, in many instances, the countries present a spectrum or mixture of forms rather than being totally distinct models.

But community involvement cannot be dictated. If people do not have an understanding of

---

Examples of models

- Decentralized local government model.
- Decentralized self-managing communities of interest model.
- Pluralist public/private and elective/appointed participation model.
- Publicly regulated, autonomous organizations model.
- National political party/government/mass movement interactive model.

---

the roles they can play, or where the culture and attitudes of health professionals and other personnel are not supportive of their efforts, community participation will be no more than a catch phrase. Nor can community involvement survive only on the energies of individuals at that level.

For community involvement to be effective, certain prerequisites are necessary. A clear national policy is needed, to encourage community cohesion in health-promotion efforts. Some other measures will further promote community involvement such as: a national commitment to support community involvement; decentralization with delegation of responsibility and authority and accountability; development of local structures; creation of different community health bodies fostering individual responsibility for self care; ensuring the representation of the people at the highest level of decision-making; intersectoral cooperation; good communication within and outside the community; logistic support; and involvement of nongovernmental organizations.

A large majority of Member States consider community involvement not only a political necessity but also an important and effective mechanism for planning, implementing and evaluating health programmes. Of the 151 country reports so far reviewed, 94 stated that mechanisms are fully functioning or being further developed, 7 replied negatively, and in 50 reports

no information was given (see Annex table: global indicator 2).

One of the countries in which the mechanism is fully functioning is Finland, where an increasing demand and willingness of people to have a say in matters that concern their health is matched with social demand and community priorities.

The following explanations were given by countries which replied that community involvement is not functioning: the mechanism is being restructured (Argentina); community involvement in health care has yet to be established (Bangladesh); numerous organs do ensure community involvement (Central African Republic); and the problem is not yet clear (Namibia).

Some countries reported that it is difficult to mobilize communities to participate in health activities, mainly because of excessive centralization in the control of resources and decision-making and lack of clear ideas of what communities should be expected to do.

Some of the developing countries have mechanisms for involving people in the implementation of health-for-all strategies that are fully functioning; others are in the process of being further developed. As to community involvement, experience to date suggests that there are a number of basic principles which are the key to the successful establishment and functioning of such mechanisms (6). These include:

- a partnership between health services and their professionals and local community people;
- individual and collective leadership at the community level; and
- sustainable mechanisms at the community level.

A number of countries are gradually beginning to recognize the important role of nongovernmental organizations in linking the community with the health system and other sectors. There is growing awareness and wider acceptance of the role played by these organizations in health activities. However, clear political commitment and effective strategies are required to harness these resources. Several countries have initiated consultation and cooperation at national, provincial, and local levels. A number of successful initiatives and projects in different parts of the world demonstrate the value of the partnership approach. In some countries in Asia, national nongovernmental organizations have formed associations to offer advice and support in the implementation of national plans. Individually and collectively they undertake primary health care activities, provide managerial support to smaller organizations, and cooperate with the ministries of health in various programme areas. In a few countries, federations of nongovernmental organizations collaborate in official programmes. Examples of their work are found in specific disease-oriented activities such as malaria control, immunization campaigns, and blindness prevention, as well as in programmes for the elderly or for handicapped persons, and in health promotion activities such as family planning and anti-smoking campaigns. Yet the absence of a policy framework for coordinating these efforts is a significant obstacle.

In Africa, communities are becoming involved through the district to which they belong. This requires enhancement of their capabilities, properly functioning community health committees, and supervisory district health and developmental committees. In July 1990, people-to-people cooperation by the special Health Fund for Africa was launched in Addis Ababa, with the objective of linking communities with their counterparts in other African countries and other regions.

All Middle East countries reported that mechanisms for involving people are fully functioning or being further developed; however, they mentioned that the lack of a clear role is also common. The role played by nongovernmental organizations varies here: it may be at a high level in planning (Pakistan), or more often of a practical nature such as promoting blood donation (Cyprus) or health education and "health weeks" (Saudi Arabia).

Algeria reports the creation of an impressive number of health-related associations and patient groups, especially since 1988. At different levels, political and other groups participate actively in health councils and management committees.

To increase community awareness of health problems at all levels, in some countries of south-east Asia such as India, in addition to the training of health personnel in community mobilization and organization, the training for opinion leaders has been organized, village health committees have been formed, and voluntary and nongovernmental organizations have been invited to participate in health services projects.

In some countries, community involvement in health development is identified as the main strategy to achieve the objective of extending health care to all villages through a village self-managed primary health care programme, while other community development schemes have fostered a closer community spirit.

Community health workers also play an important role in stimulating and supporting community initiatives, and in linking the community to other sectors and levels of the health system. In Thailand, village health communicators and village health volunteers are motivators of community involvement and are involved in programme development in addition to their service functions. In Indonesia, the community health worker's role in linking the community to the health sector is stressed. In Mozambique, community health workers are active in all aspects of health work and community mobilization for development.

In many of the South Pacific island countries, the traditional system of collective responsibility remains vital to the effective organization of community services. This is seen most notably in Fiji (see box). This system is also considered effective for promoting healthy habits and life styles.

Community involvement in Fiji

The Vulowai Health Committee of Fiji is a voluntary nongovernmental organization established in 1985 to implement the principles of primary health care in an underprivileged rural setting. Monthly meetings and village inspections are held with active community participation. The main activities of the Committee include self-help projects – a community pharmacy, water-sealed latrines, and the building of an access road to the health centre. The location of the monthly meetings is decided on a rotation basis, thus ensuring that no village is overlooked. Apart from the presence of teams from the Ministry of Health as professional advisers, the inspections and discussions are the full responsibility of the community.

The majority of least developed countries are trying to further develop or improve already existing mechanisms for community involvement. Many countries lack personnel trained in the art of communication, education, and stimulation of community development, but more involvement of nongovernmental organizations and the development of community revolving cooperative schemes are recent trends in some least developed countries. In Nepal a community health volunteer scheme launched in the districts, drawing upon the self-help potential of the community, has helped generate community involvement and strengthen programme implementation.

Member countries from the Americas reported that the diversity of mechanisms established for community participation reflects the diversity of the national sociopolitical contexts.

Vaccination campaigns and the involvement of nongovernmental organizations were mentioned as successful examples of community participation.

The trend in some western European countries is for people to be more willing to have a say in matters that concern their health and medical care, indeed even to demand it, but only a few governments are able or willing to exploit this trend to create additional mechanisms for community involvement. In central and eastern European countries it is rather the opposite, with governments now very keen to establish new structures to allow for more real community participation, while people are still hesitant.

During the 1980s there were numerous and varied developments in western Europe in respect of life styles and health behaviour, and most progress was made in the area of self-help, self-care, and local health initiative groups such as the noncommunicable diseases integrated programme approach in Austria. The evidence for increased action at the local level comes from the feedback on the success of the WHO Healthy Cities Project (7). The aim of the project was to put health higher on the agenda of city policies. It turned into the European healthy cities movement, which already counts hundreds of self-help groups involving 30 initial project cities, with 500 more cities (in 18 European countries) in the process of joining in and a clear trend towards further growth. This fast-growing movement is often based on nongovernmental organizations, including patient and consumer groups. The overall self-help movement in Europe is reaching a level of progress which matches the expectations set for this target in the early 1980s.

The quantity and quality of educational programmes to enhance the knowledge, motivation and skills of people to acquire and maintain health has steadily increased in the past 10 years in all western European countries. Numerous health education activities have been carried out by national, regional and local governments as well as by a variety of nongovernmental organizations. Major areas of concern are tobacco, alcohol, drugs, infectious and noncommunicable diseases, nutrition, physical activity, sports injuries, school health, care of the elderly and disabled, safety of consumer goods, accident prevention and road safety, worksite nutrition and catering management, human relations and sexuality, AIDS, the humanization of health care, and the promotion of social security. There is a growing tendency to fight against emerging health problems by using the health advocacy/promotion approach by well-recognized and well-organized intersectoral groups, as in Denmark.

The picture is less favourable for central and eastern European countries, which are in the process of reorganizing their basic health education and health promotion infrastructures. They sometimes experience increasing difficulties in getting the basic material for publications, let alone money for audiovisual aids or for evaluation measures. Hungary created a national institute for health promotion, and Czechoslovakia and Poland are in the process of doing so.

Two important obstacles have emerged in achieving progress in community involvement: the absence of clear national policies or strategies for the establishment of community health worker programmes and the lack of specific and regular budgetary support from governments to sustain training, supervision, logistics, and financial incentives, which are important factors in the success of these programmes.

Sometimes obstacles are caused by centralized administrative structures or rigidly organized health systems. Other problems may arise from professional staff who fear loss of their control and power, or from members of the public, who may think that someone is already paid to do the job. The most frequently mentioned problems in the least developed countries are: the low level of general education, lack of knowledge about diseases, and the absence of clear mechanisms for involving people.

Supporting legislation

Legislation is one of the key mechanisms for supporting health policies and programmes and for regulating the activities of the health system. Other mechanisms are discussed in chapter 4.

The importance of legislation in support of health development was clearly recognized by Member States during the preparation of their national strategies for health for all. It is generally recognized that such an ambitious goal as health for all cannot be achieved in the absence of an up-to-date, enlightened, and realistic framework of laws, regulations, and other instruments that make clear the responsibilities of the state, other national and subnational authorities, members of the health professions, and the different elements of society concerned with health development.

Health legislation can be used in a variety of areas, in addition to supporting national health policies and strategies:

(1) to support basic human rights (including the right to health, patients' rights, issues related to discrimination);

(2) to support changes in the health system and in health care financing and manpower development;

(3) to support environmental health policies;

(4) to promote healthy life styles (e.g., by anti-tobacco legislation) and ensure that consumer goods meet prescribed safety standards; and

(5) to support and control new technologies (reproduction, genetics, organ replacement, etc.).

In recent years, many Member States have reviewed their existing health laws and regulations with a view to supporting health development, reorienting health systems towards the primary health care approach, improving the quality of the human environment, and combating health-damaging behavioural patterns (smoking and other forms of substance abuse), all of which are important for improving health and achieving the goal of health for all by the year 2000.

Recently developments in legislation in some developed countries (e.g., Finland, Luxembourg, and Switzerland) have paid particular attention to the disabled, and specifically their social and occupational rehabilitation. These laws cover the mentally disabled in some countries. However, other countries (e.g., Denmark and Sweden) prefer to avoid special legislation for the disabled and focus more on developing self-help programmes. Progress has also been made in the introduction of legal and administrative measures for health protection, the prevention of health-damaging behaviour, and the promotion of positive health behaviour. A good example in the case of tobacco policies is Finland, which introduced measures for the restriction of tobacco smoking in 1977, later followed by many other countries.

Manufacturers and importers are now accepting greater responsibility for damage to health caused by their products, usually as a result of pressure on the part of the public. In Sweden, it is now possible to demand complete withdrawal of harmful products from the market. This is also the case in Finland, where a new Product Safety Act was passed by Parliament in June 1990.

Political pressures have now reached a level that allows ministries of health to reduce health-damaging behaviour in the northern and western European countries, mainly in connection with tobacco and alcohol. There is a move towards a total ban on tobacco advertising and other forms of sales promotion.

The importance of legislative support for health development has been recognized by almost all the developing countries (including the least developed countries), and different activities have been launched to develop, modify, and update existing health legislation to implement national health policies for health for all by the year 2000.

Realizing the importance of having well-defined and updated health legislation to implement their national strategies, eight Middle Eastern countries have reviewed their health laws and regulations in the period since the first evaluation was undertaken in 1985. The thrust of the reforms has been towards the reorganization of health services and/or the ministry of health (strengthening the planning process, decentralization, regionalization, etc.).

Many Far Eastern and Pacific countries periodically review their legislation, particularly that in the field of public health and the practice of the health professions. The aim is to reflect new technology, ideas, and practices or to provide for the registration of certain categories of health personnel (e.g., Malaysia). China has engaged in activities designed to raise awareness among managers concerning the use of health legislation.

In some developing countries, legislation has been enacted to provide health services for the entire population (e.g., Mongolia), while in others emphasis has been placed on legislation dealing with health manpower (Indonesia). In one of the Indian States (Maharashtra), legislation is pending that would prohibit commercial trafficking in human organs for transplantation purposes.

In some least developed countries, amendments were made to the law to bring it into line with new health policies (Myanmar); an Act was passed in Nepal to support the decentralization of health delivery systems, while in Bangladesh improved health laws were drafted and pioneering drug policy legislation enacted.

Experience so far in the development and implementation of health legislation indicates that legislators should now begin to look more to health legislation to support the comprehensive provision of primary health care, instead of the implementation of its isolated elements.

Intercountry cooperation

Generally, there is a progressive trend in cooperation among countries which includes increased intercountry dialogue, information exchange, study tours to meet specific needs, training, health systems research, and also other areas such as malaria, nutrition, and pharmaceuticals. The following tendencies were noted recently:

- developed countries are more in favour of direct cooperation with recipient countries; and
- developing and least developed countries are making an effort to revise priority areas for cooperation.

For example, the Far Eastern, Pacific, and south-east Asian countries mentioned positive cooperation among themselves as well as with other developing and developed countries for health development.

Though countries note progress, most appear to believe that the great potential for cooperation is yet to be realized. For instance, intercountry discussion and dialogue does not always lead to useful projects.

A few countries in the Americas have systematically analysed their needs for external cooperation and most of them have established bilateral agreements with neighbouring countries, especially to deal with communicable diseases of common interest.

Intercountry cooperation is considered satisfactory by Member States in Africa. The main subjects for cooperation are: exchange of experiences and information, especially for epidemics and common training programmes.

Some geopolitical organizations (ASEAN and SAARC) have enabled Asian countries to cooperate among themselves, but more on a bilateral basis. There is also a tendency to cooperate more closely with immediate neighbours. Thailand has extended its cooperation in the areas of PHC and health manpower development, not only to south-east Asian countries, but also to Middle Eastern countries.

Although the potential for technical cooperation among developing countries (TCDC) is considered by countries as high, there has not been a consistent approach to TCDC by some developing countries (in south-east Asia) mainly owing to a lack of sustained support to bring developing countries together and to a lack of continuing support for the organizations dealing with TCDC. Financing of TCDC is one of the problems. Funds to bring countries together are often very limited.

In many intercountry projects, there are perennial problems of poor coordination between the parties involved, particularly in programme planning (Far Eastern and Pacific countries). Part of the reason for only limited success is that many cooperation agencies do not have appropriate budget lines for technical exchange, which means that funding specifically for technical cooperation is not forthcoming.

Some selective cooperation also exists among countries on such topics as fellowships, district health systems, healthy cities, and health learning materials, with WHO playing a catalytic role.

External assistance has been an important source of financial support, complementing national health budgets in many developing and least developed countries. The majority of these countries will need continued support through collaborative programmes carried out by bilateral and multilateral agencies. Countries have taken important steps to sustain as well as further strengthen international cooperation in health by undertaking procedural adjustments, setting up new coordination mechanisms and improving capacity for the efficient management of resources.

Cooperation with WHO and other agencies

International action to support the implementation of national strategies is one of the prerequisites for achieving the goal of health for all. The majority of Member States reporting on international cooperation mentioned "cordial", "productive", and "close" collaboration with WHO. A number of countries have established committees or other mechanisms for monitoring and coordinating the implementation of joint WHO/ country collaborative programmes. They also reported improved collaboration with WHO over the past few years. Most of this improvement appears to be the result of initiatives from the countries themselves, which have become more actively involved in preparing programmes of collaboration with WHO. Sometimes it has arisen through WHO's further involvement in country activities calling for monitoring and coordination for efficient implementation. An exchange of views between countries and regional offices is undertaken in a number of different ways: at the regional committees and subcommittees, through joint government/WHO programme review missions, and in meetings in the regional office attended by the WHO representatives.

The main thrust of WHO collaboration in Member countries was focused on joint collaborative programmes consolidating the gains already made and addressing problems and constraints previously identified, to accelerate the process of implementation. WHO has continued to promote collaboration between countries and recognized nongovernmental organizations in support of health development in those countries. This includes both national ones and those from outside the country or region. WHO has established a partnership with ministries of health, planning, and finance, and other ministries related to health, to ensure that the health sector is developed within broader national socioeconomic development priorities.

WHO representatives play a crucial role in the successful implementation of WHO's collaborative programmes at country level. In addition to technical support provided by WHO staff and consultants to the countries in the implementation of country activities, other forms of WHO collaboration with the countries were intercountry/regional meetings and consultations, increased exchange of information, monitoring and evaluation of different programmes and projects, and the provision of fellowships in the relevant areas. WHO collaborated with Member States in their efforts to develop TCDC in the field of health, by providing catalytic financial support to the concerned sectors in organizations such as SAARC and ASEAN.

Countries are considering their health structures, approaches and resources with a view to adjusting or reorienting them as a part of their economic adjustment policies. They are making sustained efforts to improve and strengthen their national health systems based on primary health care. Careful attention has been paid to the way health resources should be used, with a view to reallocating them in the context of the countries' macroeconomic adjustment policies.

The main issues that countries have faced in this endeavour have been the need to build up a capacity to coordinate aid agencies, the need to direct support towards sustainable health development, and the need to include health components in all development projects. International cooperation, often time-limited and focused on selective health development components, has not always been able to give countries the means for independent and sustained development. Both countries and development agencies have realized the need to improve the efficiency of their cooperation. In many countries, cooperation policies are being formulated and mechanisms developed.

In 1989, to assist in further health development and to help overcome difficulties, WHO launched a new strategy of intensified cooperation with countries and peoples in greatest need. Frameworks for collaborative action have been set up in each participating country, including the more efficient use of the country's own resources and the expansion of the role played in the coordination of resources mobilized from the international community. This strategy aims at focusing all existing resources into coherent and coordinated action, country by country, through all WHO's programmes, and at all levels of the Organization, in conjunction with all the existing or potential energies and resources of international cooperation.

So far, 20 countries have collaborated in WHO's intensified cooperation initiatives, with the support of the main intergovernmental and official development assistance agencies. Various partnership arrangements have been developed between countries, WHO, and development agencies. Pragmatic national action plans, developed in countries with the support of WHO, now provide the main frameworks for improved coordination and better resource allocation to health.

One Country: Guinea-Bissau

The Government of Guinea-Bissau has identified three strategic lines of action for health development: the provision of essential drugs; the improvement of health infrastructures, and the training of health manpower personnel. In addition, other areas needing support are the establishment of an epidemiological surveillance system and the development of a malaria control plan. A national document has been prepared and will serve as the health sector input for the UNDP programming cycle meeting.

International support to selected areas (such as health finance), and studies carried out by the World Bank, WHO and other agencies should further contribute to establishing an appropriate framework for effective cost-sharing mechanisms in the health sector, and should strengthen the planning capacity of the Ministry of Health, to increase the performance of the health system.

Countries have also promoted extensive collaboration with United Nations agencies, such as UNDP, UNICEF, and UNFPA, and also with the development banks, and a number of international NGOs. For example, a nongovernmental organization group on primary health care is working in six countries of southern Africa with WHO and UNICEF support: it has prepared a plan to promote collaboration with Botswana, Lesotho, Malawi, Swaziland, Zambia, and Zimbabwe in planning, implementing and reviewing public health care programmes. The technical cooperation programmes with these agencies have provided considerable support to national initiatives across diverse areas of health development.

Some concern was expressed by countries in the Far East and Pacific about cooperation between agencies working in the same countries, particularly in the case of smaller countries. It was mentioned that agencies usually exchange information on their plans and achievements, but at the implementation stage duplication is often hard to avoid. More efficient use of resources would be achieved if cooperation between agencies was made early in the planning stage of an activity.

Summary and conclusions

From the very beginning health for all by the year 2000 as a social goal, although unanimously accepted by all Member States of WHO, created more curiosity than a real intention for its implementation. The question asked by everyone was: what is it? and not: how can it be done?

As time passed, decision-makers became more aware of the potential of health for all for improving health status and for decreasing inequalities. Of course, doubts have always been present, especially after realizing that on the way to achieving it many problems and constraints existed. If Member States had considered at the time only the problems and constraints, and not the possibilities and opportunities, they might not have defined the policies and adopted such ambitious goals.

Thirteen years after Alma-Ata and with the experience of several monitoring and evaluation exercises, questions such as "what is it?" were no longer relevant.

The main emphasis of the first evaluation of the strategy for health for all in 1985 was on the assessment of the situation and processes, and their compatibility with the principles of the strategy. The second evaluation concentrates on evaluating progress in the implementation of the strategy with a view to knowing: (1) what has been implemented; (2) how far it has contributed to the progress of implementation of the strategy; and (3) what were the critical impediments at national, regional, and global levels. The focus has been on those areas that can truly reflect progress in relation to the health-for-all strategy in totality, and not on various elements of primary health care.

In relation to health policies and strategies, it is clear now that in most countries, health-for-all policy and goals have continued to receive endorsement. National health policies and plans of action to achieve these goals have been formulated, adjusted, or revised in response to changes in the political and socioeconomic environment; laws have also been reviewed or revised as necessary to support national health policies and strategies. Following increased understanding of the principles of health for all and primary health care, initiatives to reduce inequity have been launched, usually directed to specific vulnerable groups and/or to priority health problems. Infrastructure and quality of care have been given increasing attention during the development of health systems based on primary health care. The main characteristics of health system development by level of development are shown in Table 2.1.

In order to achieve the goals of health for all, virtually all Member States have made efforts to implement the strategy through primary health care by promoting:

(1) improved access to health care and reallocation of resources towards primary health care;
(2) the integration of health services;
(3) the decentralization of responsibility and authority to the lower levels of the health system; and
(4) the involvement of communities, families, individuals, and local nongovernmental organizations as well as health personnel.

However, insufficient understanding of the basic principles of health for all, special interests and swinging priorities of decision-makers and planners, external pressure from funding agencies in some cases, lack of funds to run institutions and programmes, and resistance from some professional and interest groups to the primary health care approach have inhibited a faster pace of progress in implementing primary health care, particularly with respect to strengthening the health system infrastructure and management, especially at the peripheral level, and distributing health personnel appropriately. In some countries emphasis continues to be placed on curative services rather than on providing curative services in association with promotive and preventive care.

The major challenge faced by countries – be they developing, least developed, or developed – is to face squarely the confrontations and conflicts that are inevitable in carrying out activities in pursuit of improving health with equity; it will be necessary to mobilize collaboration and direct partnership with communities and other partners (professionals and other pressure groups and other agencies and organizations). The direction taken by most Member States appears to be: to further develop and strengthen health infrastructures with community involvement; to provide comprehensive health care through integrated services and activities; to support intersectoral coordination for effectiveness and efficiency; to ensure the quality of care given; and to sustain what has already been achieved.

Table 2.1
Health system development: main characteristics by level of development

Subject/content	Developing countries	Least developed countries	Developed countries	Eastern European countries
1. Health policies and strategies	Majority formulated national health policies and committed to implementation	Majority formulated national health policies and committed to implementation	Majority formulated national health policies and committed to implementation	Majority of formulated national health policies being revised and adjusted to new political environment
1.1 Endorsement of HFA policy	HFA continues to receive endorsement at highest level	In a few, HFA not yet formally endorsed HFA continues to receive endorsement at highest level, but not fully followed by implementation	HFA continues to receive endorsement at highest level	Progress in implementation slowed due to political, social and economic changes
1.2 Equity	Equity important issue in health policies; efforts to establish more equity between different population groups (underprivileged)	Equity important issue in health policies; emphasis on equity in health status, rural, urban slums, vulnerable groups, etc.	Equity recognized as important objective of HFA; targets to reduce inequities set by majority; emphasis on disadvantaged national groups	Equity important issue; some vulnerable groups and areas identified for special support
1.3 Allocation and distribution of resources for PHC	Resources for PHC being distributed towards rural populations/areas; still some differences between population groups/programmes	Resources for PHC being distributed towards rural populations/areas; still some differences between population groups/programmes; very rarely, no change in distribution	Resources for PHC evenly distributed to all regions/provinces	
2. Organization of health systems based on PHC	Majority trying to further reorient health system towards PHC PHC accepted and expanded Steps taken towards decentralization Some have slow progress from vertical to integrated approach and explosion of expensive technology in private services	Majority accepted PHC and trying to expand Degree of understanding of PHC varies Tendency towards decentralization Health system infrastructure unsatisfactory, weak management at operational level	Majority trying to further reorient health system towards PHC PHC fully understood, accepted and expanded Decentralization being implemented Special attention to specific strategies (elderly, disabled) and need for basic reallocation of resources. Cost of health services for some population groups considered very high	Reorientation and restructuring of health system based on PHC under way based on recent introduction of health reforms in some
3. Managerial process and mechanisms	Almost all reviewed planning process and trying to strengthen plans	Measures for improvement of existing system taken in some and efforts to implement some changes in a few Lack of trained staff and inadequate health information systems	Although permanent mechanisms not always established, management not considered "weak" point in health system	Positive changes in managerial process key element in recently introduced health reforms
4. Community involvement and health promotion	Community involvement considered important and effective mechanism for implementation of HFA strategy In half, community involvement fully functioning and in half being further developed using various mechanisms	Community involvement being further developed and improved using various mechanisms In a few, not further developed	Community involvement considered important and effective mechanism for implementing HFA strategy Full responsibility of community and extensive involvement Health education and health promotion infrastructure strengthened Establishment of formal mechanism for community involvement in some	Community involvement shifting from formal political mechanism to informal self-help groups or through Red Cross or church Some health education and health promotion measures slowed down
5. Supporting legislation	Importance of supporting legislation in health development recognized Revisions made to support HFA2000 in some	Importance of supporting legislation in health development recognized Review and revision of existing laws to support national health policies in some	Legislation extended to cover more disadvantaged groups for social and occupational reintegration	Legislative support and administrative measures to promote healthy lifestyles increasing
6. Intercountry cooperation	New areas/priorities identified. Very active cooperation through ASEAN, SAARC, TCDC, etc. Selective cooperation (fellowships, etc.) Cooperation with international NGOs	Revision of priority areas; external assistance important source of financial support; tendency to improve cooperation with neighbours Cooperation with international NGOs	Well established international cooperation Tendency to cooperate directly with recipient countries	Due to recent political changes, international cooperation is under review
7. Cooperation with WHO and other agencies	Productive/close and even cordial with WHO For some, international aid insignificant compared to national resources	Productive/close and cordial with WHO Satisfied with large number of donors	Very satisfactory Tendency to cooperate directly with recipient countries	Very satisfactory

Source: Based on national and regional evaluation reports.

References

1. *Global strategy for health for all by the year 2000*. Geneva, World Health Organization, 1981 ("Health for All" Series, No. 3).

2. *From Alma-Ata to the year 2000: reflections at the midpoint*. Geneva, World Health Organization, 1988; and *Alma-Ata reaffirmed at Riga*. Geneva, World Health Organization, 1988 (document WHA41/1988/REC/1).

3. *Alma-Ata 1978: primary health care*. Geneva, World Health Organization, 1978 ("Health for All" Series, No. 1).

4. *Glossary of terms used in the "Health for All" series, No. 1-8*. Geneva, World Health Organization, 1984 ("Health for All" Series, No. 9).

5. *Managerial process for national health development: guiding principles*. Geneva, World Health Organization, 1981 ("Health for All" Series, No. 5).

6. *People-to-people cooperation: a framework based on Africa's health scenario*. Brazzaville, WHO Regional Office for Africa, 1991.

7. *Healthy cities project: a project becomes a movement: review of progress, 1987 and 1990*. Copenhagen, WHO Regional Office for Europe, 1991.

CHAPTER 3
Health care

Introduction

Since the first evaluation of the implementation of the health-for-all strategies in 1985 there have been substantial developments in the coverage of populations with health care. These changes result from various factors. Most notable is the extent of government, political and social commitment to achieving HFA. The commitment of financial resources for health by governments and the mobilization of resources by individuals and communities themselves is another essential factor along with growing management capabilities for programme implementation both among health personnel and at community level. Health personnel are better trained and oriented to communicating and working more effectively with their peers, with government, with other sectors, and with individuals and communities. The decentralization of planning, decision-making, and financial authority to lower levels and much greater community involvement in local health planning and decision-making have been very important ingredients too. There is also the growing availability of affordable, simple, and effective health technologies that can be readily obtained by and used at community level.

In spite of these developments, many problems remain. The percentage of the population covered with essential services has increased, but millions of people remain without access to water and sanitation services and to the basic elements of care because the increases in services available have not kept pace with the increases in population. The gap between the availability of different elements of health care in developed countries and in the least developed countries is widening, even though there are clearly improvements globally, even in the poorest group of countries. There are also wide gaps within countries, between rich and poor and even between different parts of big cities, often made worse by the economic decline of the 1980s. Services are often fragmented; developed as well as developing countries report the need for improved coordination between the public and private sectors and with nongovernmental organizations.

In some countries second- and third-level health care are not well developed. The lack of possibilities for first-level providers to get advice and information from higher levels, and thereby avoid the need to refer certain problems to higher levels, and the lack of possibility where needed of referring complicated problems or emergencies for additional specialized or technically complex care, can have major consequences for the health and well-being of patients and their families. It can also contribute to a loss of credibility for health providers and the health system. Where highly specialized and/or costly third-level care is given the greatest priority, this can contribute to inadequate care for the most common problems affecting the majority of the people. The quality of care is generally high in most developed countries, although the overavailability of drugs and of technology, which is often more complex than the situation calls for, lead to other kinds of problems. In many developing countries the quality of care, equipment, and drugs is often much lower than in other parts of the world.

This chapter sketches overall trends in the development of health care during the period 1985-1990 and highlights some of the specific trends revealed by information from countries for coverage with the different subelements of global indicator 7 (see box).

Indicator 7 does not require countries to provide information on the extent of coverage with *all* the named elements or subelements of the indicator. Rather, countries are requested to indicate the extent of coverage for the various subelements, and this is the information reflected in Fig. 3.1-3.10. The chapter also provides information on issues not specifically covered by global indicator 7, in order to give a fuller picture of the many other developments in health care that have taken place in countries in response to the many health challenges they now face. In order to emphasize the interrelationship between the various subelements of

---

Global indicator 7

The percentage of the population covered by primary health care, with at least the following:

- safe water in the home or with reasonable access and with adequate excreta-disposal facilities available;

- immunization against diphtheria, tetanus, whooping-cough, measles, poliomyelitis, and tuberculosis;

- local health services, including availability of essentiel drugs, within one hour's walk or travel;

- attendance by trained personnel for pregnancy and childbirth, and caring for children up to at least 1 year of age.

The percentage of women of childbearing age using family planning.

---

care referred to in this chapter and their synergistic contributions to improving health status, information is not addressed separately according to the subelements of indicator 7. The chapter begins with information on the first element referred to in the indicator, which in turn has two subelements, namely safe water and sanitation.

It is also important to be aware before reading this chapter that primary health care has several meanings – each of which is complementary to the other.

Primary health care can be looked at:

- as a range of programmes adapted to the patterns of health and disease of people living in a particular setting;

- as a level of care (the exact definition depending upon the country concerned) backed up by a well-organized referral system;

- as a strategy for reorienting the health system in order to provide the whole population with effective essential care, and to promote individual and community involvement and intersectoral collaboration; and

- as a philosophy, based on the principles of social equity, self-reliance, and community development (*1*).

The focus of this chapter is on health services and health care at the first level of contact with the health system. To avoid confusion between at least two of the definitions given above, reference in this chapter will be to the "first level of care", and to specific elements of care.

Safe water supply and sanitation

The availability of safe water and adequate sanitation continues to increase overall, although millions of people in the developing countries still do not have access to safe water supply and adequate sanitation. Nothing makes clearer the precariousness of this situation and the potentially disastrous impact on health and on national economies of such inadequacies as the spread of cholera in the 1990s to the Americas – a region which had been free of the disease for almost a century. In a number of African countries too, cholera cases are increasing at a catastrophic pace.

It is estimated that the recent outbreak of cholera could cost the impoverished economy of Peru, alone, up to US$ 1 billion in 1991 as a result of reduced economic activity, losses in the fishing, agriculture and tourism sectors, unemployment, reduction of exports, and general health infrastructure costs. The interrelationship between health and development and between national and international health issues is clearly shown in the cholera outbreak, which will in both the short and long term have a negative impact on national economic development, which in turn will have adverse consequences for health and thereby start a vicious circle.

Population coverage for safe water supply has increased from 68% in 1985 to 75% in 1991, while for adequate excreta disposal, coverage increased from 46% to 71% (see Annex table, global indicators 7.1 and 7.2). Fig. 3.1 and 3.2

respectively show coverage rates for safe water supplies and sanitation facilities for 1991 in comparison to 1985. These figures show that improvements have been made but do not make it clear that the lack of clean water remains acute for many millions of people. A more detailed look at the global situation is provided in chapter 6.

Although globally by 1990, safe water supplies had been extended to 81% of urban dwellers and 58% of rural inhabitants, and adequate sanitation coverage was 71% in urban and 48% in rural areas, 1500 million people still lack access to clean water supplies, and 2000 million still live without adequate sanitation. Despite increases in the percentage of people supplied with safe water and adequate sanitation, growing numbers of people still remain without access to these basic services due to population increase.

In terms of relative need, Africa has the lowest rate of water coverage (44%), while south-east Asia has the lowest sanitation coverage (20%). In absolute terms, however, the needs are greatest among the countries of south-east Asia, where more than 400 million

Fig. 3.1
Safe water: population coverage (global indicator 7.1), 1985 and 1991

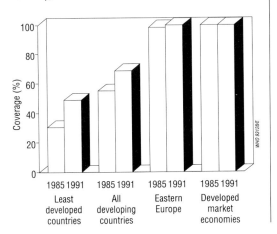

Fig. 3.2
Adequate excreta-disposal facilities: population coverage (global indicator 7.2), 1985 and 1991

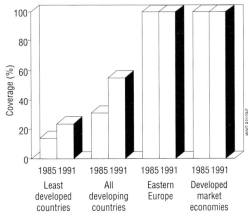

people lack safe water supply and over 1000 million remain without adequate sanitation coverage.

Increasingly, the provision of water for personal hygiene is considered just as important to health as the provision of safe water for drinking and cooking. Thus, the focus is shifting from drinking-water quality alone to one of overall environmental improvement involving water supplies, sanitation, hygiene education, the safe disposal of used water and general community involvement in environmental management. The impact of this more holistic approach can be seen in the dramatic progress in controlling dracunculiasis – a parasitic disease transmitted solely by contaminated drinking-water. Between 1985 and 1990, global incidence fell from over 10 million cases to 3 million, a drop entirely attributable to incorporating into primary health care such simple and inexpensive measures as the straining of all drinking-water to remove the vector and measures to prevent contamination of clean water sources. Global eradication of this disease is technically feasible given appropriate political, social, and economic support; in May 1991 the World Health Assembly adopted resolution WHA44.5 calling for the eradication of dracunculiasis by 1995.

Care for mothers and children

This element is covered at length both because much information is available and because developments in maternal and child care speak volumes about a country's commitment to and progress towards equity in health.

Care for mothers

Every day the equivalent of four jumbo jet planes full of women die from complications of pregnancy and childbirth. This adds up to half a million deaths a year, most of them in developing countries – as is more fully described in chapter 5. However, even in the world's most de-

veloped countries, there are some women who start pregnancy unhealthy or malnourished and anaemic, who lack access to effective family planning and who do not have sufficient care (or care of adequate quality) during pregnancy or childbirth.

Maternal mortality is an indicator of women's status in society and of their access to health care and other essential services. Inadequate care during pregnancy and childbirth, including inadequate referral to higher levels of care when required, inappropriate timing and spacing of pregnancies, and excessive numbers of pregnancies, as well as poor health and nutritional status before ever becoming pregnant, are responsible for most maternal deaths, for much infant mortality, and for a great deal of serious morbidity among women and their children.

As a result of maternal deaths, 1 million children become motherless each year, and many of them die soon after. Many millions of women develop urinary incontinence, uterine prolapse, and fistulas as a result of poor care, or no care by trained personnel during delivery. These conditions in turn contribute to chronic infections and ill health, in turn placing additional burdens on health services and adding to the cycle of maternal and child mortality and morbidity. Repeated pregnancies in already malnourished women worsen their nutritional status and contributes to chronic anaemia.

That this level of maternal mortality and morbidity persists year after year despite the increase in the availability of trained personnel to care for pregnant women (see Fig. 3.3) and the improvements in coverage by trained personnel for deliveries (see Fig. 3.4) is truly the "scandal of modern times" that it has been dubbed. It is also evidence of persisting grave inequalities in access to the health services that do exist, in living standards and in social status between countries and between groups within countries, and in female literacy and educational levels. The disparity between maternal death rates in developing countries and those in developed coun-

Fig. 3.3

Prenatal care: coverage by trained personnel (global indicator 7.6), 1985 and 1991

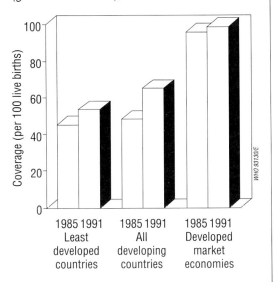

Fig. 3.4

Childbirth attendance: coverage by trained personnel (global indicator 7.7), 1985 and 1991

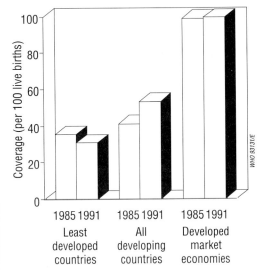

tries is greater than for any other common cause of death.

In developed countries, 99% of deliveries are performed by personnel who are usually very highly trained and who have access to equipment – much of which is more sophisticated than required for the majority of deliveries – and who can readily refer complicated pregnancies or emergencies to even more specialized services. In contrast, in some developing countries, less than 20% of deliveries are attended by trained personnel, many of whom are trained not as physicians and nurses but as birth attendants to handle the most common needs – that is, routine and uncomplicated deliveries. Facilities for referring emergencies and complicated deliveries do not always exist. If they do, they are often far away, are called upon too late, are inaccessible owing to poor roads or transport problems, or are lacking in equipment, supplies, and trained personnel.

The United Nations Decade for Women (1976–1985) helped to heighten awareness of the magnitude of these problems and the realization that they cannot continue to be accepted as inevitable, because specific and feasible solutions do exist.

Egypt, Guinea, Indonesia and many other developing countries have initiated programmes and action for safe motherhood. These place particular emphasis on making maternal health services better and more widely available and on extending family planning and education.

In every socioeconomic setting, the children of literate women have a better chance of survival than those born to illiterate mothers. Women with schooling tend to marry later and to delay childbearing, and are more likely to practise family planning, to reject harmful traditional practices related to childbirth, to adopt healthy feeding habits, to see the need for immunization of themselves and their children, to have good domestic hygiene, to use available health services in times of illness, and to see the importance of education for their own children. The World Conference on Education For All in

Jomtien, Thailand, in March 1990 stressed the concept of basic education, literacy, and a range of skills and knowledge for living (2).

Family planning

The use of affordable and straightforward technologies, which are available to all women now, could substantially reduce maternal mortality. For example, family planning is a crucial element in avoiding high-risk pregnancies, including pregnancy in women under the age of 18 and after the age of 35, in spacing births at least two or three years apart and in reducing the total number of pregnancies in a woman's lifetime. From only 9% in 1960–1965, contraceptive prevalence in developing countries has risen to an estimated level of 50% in 1990.

Information on the percentage of women of child-bearing age using family planning is sparse, as can be seen from the Annex table (global indicator 7.9), and most of the data quoted refer to information from the early to mid-1980s. Meaningful conclusions cannot therefore be drawn from these data. However, a great deal of information from other sources is available. About 300 million couples who do not want any more children are not using any method of family planning, even though surveys in developing countries show that they know the risks to women's and children's health of frequent pregnancy and that they want to limit or space future births. One method of contraception, namely condoms, has the additional advantage of preventing sexually transmitted diseases. About 6000 million condoms are being used each year, although it is estimated that about twice as many are needed. The gap is not in the supply of condoms but rather in public access to, demand for, and use of condoms. Thus, current consumption falls far short of the current public health need for condoms to prevent pregnancy and disease (3). In many countries, contraceptive use is denied to unmarried women. The International Conference on Population, held in Mexico in 1984, urged governments "to take appropriate steps to help women avoid abortion which in no case should be promoted as a method of family planning ..." (4). Yet, it is estimated that as many as one-quarter to one-third of maternal deaths each year may be a consequence of the complications of unsafe abortion procedures. This makes unsafe abortion one of the great neglected problems of health care – for developed as well as for developing countries. Contrary to common belief, studies show that most women seeking abortion are married or live in stable unions and already have several children. Abortion, therefore, serves to limit family size. Despite this, unsafe abortions and their complications are not being recognized as a significant health and social problem – which could so easily be prevented – because of the controversial and complex political, social, moral, and religious issues involved (4).

In recent years a number of countries that recorded good advances in contraceptive use and consequently lower birth rates in the late 1960s or early 1970s have found further progress difficult. They include India, the Philippines, and Morocco and some countries reporting early high gains, e.g. Tunisia. In some cases, this is the result of reduced family planning efforts because of slackening political support, while in others recession and debt burdens have forced cutbacks in government spending in such areas as family planning, health, and education. Even in some developed countries, for economic and political reasons, the end of the 1980s saw a reduction in family planning services, the health consequences of which are greatest for the lowest socioeconomic groups.

The corollaries of accelerated population growth are often the uneven distribution of peoples, migration, and rapid urbanization. In combination with poverty, population growth can seriously affect natural resources including: food and water supplies; the environment; the availability of and access to health care; the global climate; and the socioeconomic fabric of na-tions. The groups most likely to first feel the ef-fects of economic downturns, of deteriorating living conditions and environmental standards and of less care and fewer services continue to be the rural and urban poor, women, children, migrants, refugees, and the aged, especially in developing countries.

Care for children

Just as maternal health is dependent on many factors, the health of newborns and children is also strongly related to the social, economic, and health status of mothers. Most infant and under-5 morbidity and mortality could be pre-vented through the provision of adequate water supplies and sanitation facilities at community level, good nutrition of mother and child, and access to first-level care including good immu-nization coverage. The Annex table (global indi-cator 7.8) shows that coverage by trained per-sonnel of infant care has increased since the first evaluation in 1985, but more importantly indi-cates the large differences that continue to exist between countries.

Even though infant and under-5 mortality rates continue to decline worldwide, 9.2 million infants still die each year in developing coun-tries. About half of these deaths occur in the neonatal period from problems related to low birth weight and prematurity – which are reflec-tions of maternal health status; from hypother-mia and birth asphyxia – which reflect the avail-ability and quality of care during delivery and immediately thereafter; and from infections – many of which are preventable by hygienic measures, including clean deliveries, and by immunization of the mothers against tetanus.

In many developing countries, over two-thirds of all paediatric admissions to hospi-tals are due to diarrhoea and pneumonia. Most of these admissions could have been avoided by early diagnosis or recognition of danger signs and by early and appropriate treatment by health

workers and/or by the families of the sick chil-dren. Each year between US$ 1 billion and US$ 2 billion are wasted on inappropriate treat-ment of diarrhoea and acute respiratory infec-tions. Virtually all developing countries have implemented programmes to reduce diarrhoea mortality and morbidity. These programmes have developed policies, strategies, targets, and plans of action, implemented as an integral part of primary health care. Correct case manage-ment at health facilities and in the home is the major emphasis, and since 1985 preventive strategies are being given increased attention, in particular the promotion of exclusive breast-feeding during the first four to six months. Evaluation of the situation has shown that, in 1989, 63% of the developing world's 1100 million children under five years of age had access to oral rehydration salts solution, compared with 50% in 1985, and that an esti-mated 36% of diarrhoea episodes were receiv-ing oral rehydration therapy compared with 18% in 1985.

Oral rehydration salts are currently pro-duced in 64 developing countries; the reported supply in 1989 was 355 million 1-litre packets of the salts or similar products globally, an in-crease from 270 million in 1985. Data reported from health facilities in 14 developing countries have shown a median decrease in admission rates of 61% and in overall case fatality rates of 71% after the introduction of oral rehydration therapy. Some hospitals observed a three-fold reduction in the percentage of diarrhoea cases receiving intravenous fluids when this therapy was introduced; such changes have had a sig-nificant impact on hospital costs.

Before 1985 the pneumonia problem in chil-dren was rarely recognized in the national health plans of developing countries, and no control programmes had been organized, except in a few Latin American countries. By 1985 WHO had formulated a global programme on acute respiratory infections; prevention of morbidity and mortality from pneumonia in children were

69

its main objectives, and standard case management was its central strategy to prevent mortality in the short term. In view of the magnitude of the problem, correct case management of acute respiratory infections was seen as essential. Technical guidelines on case management were first issued by WHO in 1985, and revised in 1988 in light of the experience with training courses and programme implementation.

The number of countries that have taken the decision to plan and implement control activities increased from seven in 1985 to 59 in 1990. Among these, 41 belonged to the group of major target countries where the infant mortality rate was greater than 40 per 1000 live births per year. Initial evaluation efforts have illustrated immediate benefits as a result of the implementation of the standard case management strategy: a dramatic reduction in the use of antibiotics and medicines for coughs and colds, a decrease in the number of cases admitted to hospital, and a shift to less expensive but equally or more effective injectable antibiotics for treatment of severe pneumonia.

Strategies for the prevention of diarrhoea, pneumonia, and many other infectious diseases of infancy and childhood include improved nutrition, particularly through improved food hygiene and exclusive breast-feeding. Exclusive breast-feeding from birth provides for health, growth, and development of the infant, and most infants require no food or fluid other than breast milk for the first 4–6 months of life to grow healthily. In addition, breast-fed babies are better protected against infections. Breast-feeding also promotes mother-child bonding, which motivates better care of the child by the mother and provides psychological wellbeing for the infant. As a supplementary advantage, a mother who fully breast-feeds with no return of menstruation has a less than 1% chance of being pregnant again in the first six months following childbirth. Immunization within the first year of life is another important component of the prevention strategy and offers a highly effective and inexpensive protection against certain very serious diseases of infancy and childhood.

Data on immunization coverage indicate that substantial increases in coverage are being made in all regions of the world. For a child to complete successfully the primary immunization series requires five separate visits and the administration of a total of eight doses of vaccine by health workers. This resulted in almost 500 million contacts in 1990. It is doubtful whether any other service provided by governments to their citizens has reached so many people, so many times in such a short period. This accomplishment is the greatest public health success story of the past decade and is one of the most significant examples of mobilizing people for a specific purpose ever undertaken. The cost of the vaccines to accomplish this was less than US$ 1 per child immunized.

A decade ago, the rate of vaccination was about 20%. It was still low in 1985 when, at a meeting commemorating the fortieth anniversary of the United Nations, the Secretary-General called for Universal Child Immunization, with a global target of 80% coverage of children under one year by 1990. Some 74 governments and more than 400 voluntary organizations supported the commitment, with the result that in 1990, on a global average 80% of all those born were successfully immunized against measles, diphtheria, pertussis, tetanus, poliomyelitis, and tuberculosis – under the Expanded Programme on Immunization of the World Health Organization and UNICEF.

By 1990, over 84% of children reaching the first year of life worldwide had been immunized with a third dose of poliomyelitis vaccine. Coverage in developing countries alone was estimated at 85% for a third dose of poliomyelitis vaccine and 83% for combined diphtheria, pertussis and tetanus (DPT) vaccine; at 90% for tuberculosis (BCG) vaccine and 79% for measles vaccine. Even so, millions of children each year do not receive these immunizations. As a result, approximately 2 million of them die. The additional tragedy is that the level of immunization of pregnant women against tetanus – which is a fundamental element of maternal care and of infant survival, and a good indicator of inequality of care – is only 39% for two or more doses of tetanus toxoid in developing countries.

Fig. 3.5–3.8 show the improvements in immunization coverage over the past six years and indicate the extent of the differences between countries in immunization coverage. The gap between the developing and developed countries has been narrowing for all the indicators; however, the increase in immunization coverage for the least developed countries has not been so fast as for the other developing countries. What these figures do not show, however, is that large differences in coverage often exist within countries, with, for example, remote rural areas or island populations having lower coverage than in the capital city and other urban centres, due to logistical problems in delivering or transporting vaccines, in maintaining the cold chain, and in maintaining the level of financial and human resources needed.

Almost all countries have adopted new disease reduction targets for diseases preventable by the EPI vaccines for the 1990s – a 90% reduction in measles compared to pre-immunization levels and elimination of neonatal tetanus by 1995 as well as the eradication of poliomyelitis by the year 2000 (World Health Assembly resolution WHA41.28). If these targets are to be achieved, however, coverage levels must not only be maintained but increased.

Experience shows that social and economic problems can constrain the ability to strengthen or to sustain immunization coverage and even jeopardize gains made to date. Sustained political commitment and financial support to immunization activities at national level are essential. Also fundamental are efforts to strengthen management, including the management of disease surveillance, laboratory services, and logistics support. Even in the most developed regions of the world, many countries report having immunization programmes with unclear targets, less than good surveillance, monitoring, and evaluation, and in some countries there are long delays in reporting outbreaks of diseases preventable by immunization.

The AIDS pandemic will have a marked impact on the type of health care and social ser-

Fig. 3.5
Immunization of infants: coverage by DPT vaccine (global indicator 7.3.2), 1985 and 1991

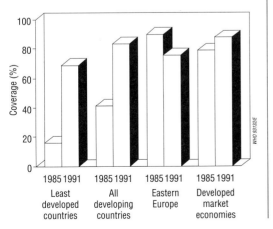

Fig. 3.6
Immunization of infants: coverage by measles vaccine (global indicator 7.3.3), 1985 and 1991

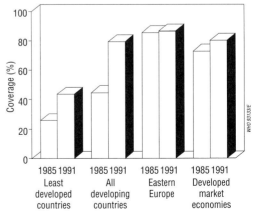

Fig. 3.7

Immunization of infants: coverage by poliomyelitis vaccine (global indicator 7.3.4), 1985 and 1991

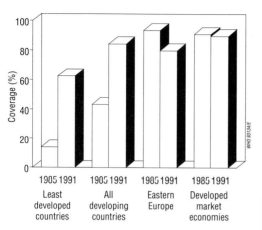

Fig. 3.8

Immunization of infants: coverage by BCG vaccine (global indicator 7.3.5), 1985 and 1991

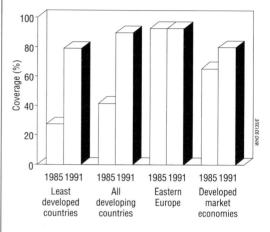

vices required for infants and children who either become infected themselves or who are left motherless.

Local health care

The data on coverage of the population with other elements of health care than those specifically referred to above are hard to interpret since the elements covered by the heading "availability of local health services" are not specified. The Annex table (global indicator 7.5) indicates the percentage of the population in different groups of countries covered by local health services. This indicator includes availability of essential drugs. More information on this subelement is given below, together with some related information on vaccines. Information on many of the other elements of care that can be assumed to be part of local health care are subsequently referred to under the heading "other health services". As reflected below, these health services range from care provided for specific health problems to preventive and promotive action, specialized care at second or third referral level, and such support services as laboratory and radiology.

There has been significant movement in recent years towards more integrated primary health care. This often stems from the disappointing results of vertical programme activities and fragmented and duplicated health care services. The objective is to make more effective use of the available health resources through integrated health care delivery and to ensure the continuity and sustainability of services. Integration of health care can involve the integration of services tasks, the integration of management and support functions, and the integration of the organizational set-up. Integration should not be limited to a single level of the health system; rather, the first-level hospital should be integrated into the district health system to facilitate referral of cases for all kinds of health needs.

Second- and third-level services are not explicitly covered because the focus of chapter 3 is on coverage at the first level of care. However, as mentioned above, the involvement of second and third levels is essential - to give back-up for preventive, promotive, curative, and rehabilitative activities, to provide care for referred patients, and to complement the skills, resources, and technical capacities of the first care level. The hospital is a partner to the other health services in the community. In addition to institutional care, hospitals give technical support and back-up to other care services, and have an important role to play in health promotion and disease prevention, diagnostic activities, rehabilitation, and the education and training of health personnel. Hospitals, therefore, need to be closely associated, along with other elements of care provided at the second and third levels, with the planning, organization, and delivery of care (5).

Availability of essential drugs and vaccines

The philosophy of the rational use of drugs is widely accepted and the concept of the essential drugs list is being implemented in many countries. Yet developing countries have problems in purchasing drugs because of their lack of foreign exchange. Moreover, based on available data, about 1000 million people seem to lack regular access to local health services.

Despite the persistence of such problems, however, there have been many notable achievements. Countries continue to adopt national drug policies which provide the basis both for rational planning at national level and for the better coordination of external technical assistance. In Bhutan, for example, the institution of a national drug plan led to a considerable increase in the availability of essential drugs over a four-year period. In Colombia, a Directorate of Health Supplies was established to give greater emphasis to the management and rational use of drugs.

In contrast to problems of undersupply, developed countries are becoming more and more aware of the magnitude of overprescribing of medicines and are increasingly concerned about the health implications, as well as about the financial strain on health services. Significant educational, research, and training efforts are under way in a number of countries including France, which has the highest per capita drug consumption in Europe, aimed at changing the prescribing habits of doctors and at changing people's habits and attitudes to the prescription and use of drugs and over-the-counter medications (6).

WHO keeps a vigilant watch over the quality of vaccines that developing countries receive through United Nations sources. Developing countries are also encouraged by WHO to apply these same standards to vaccines which are locally produced. However, many such vaccines are not up to standard. The major impact of low-quality vaccines is on infants and young children, who are most susceptible to infectious diseases, including neonatal tetanus. For example, an outbreak of diphtheria in children in one country recently may have been the result of inadequate doses of toxoid in locally produced DPT vaccines. In another country, infants suffered from neonatal tetanus even though their mothers had received a sufficient number of doses of tetanus toxoid, but it had been a low-quality vaccine from a local producer. A number of countries have taken steps to strengthen national systems for the quality control of vaccines and to give greater emphasis to the supervision and training of personnel. Not all commercially available vaccines on the international market meet WHO standards.

Other health services

Coverage at local level with a wide range of health services in addition to those referred to above continues to increase – for malaria, leprosy, or other parasitic diseases; for sexually transmitted diseases and AIDS; for tuberculosis; for common illnesses of children; for treatment of injury; for provision of eye care; for oral health care; for care of the elderly. Because of space limitations not all the different elements of those services are described below.

Leprosy. All countries where leprosy is endemic have adopted the strategy for multidrug therapy, which is cost-effective and avoids problems of drug resistance, which in turn leads to greater compliance in taking medication. By October 1990, 55.7% of all registered leprosy cases were taking this therapy. By the same date, 2 million leprosy patients were on it and 1.2 million had already completed their treatment. The increasing acceptability of this therapy for leprosy control to national health services and patients alike is due mainly to the fixed and relatively short duration of treatment, the low level of toxicity and treatment-related side-effects, and the very low relapse rates following completion of treatment. One advantage of introducing the WHO-recommended regimens is that the proportion of cases self-reporting at an early stage of the disease has increased considerably, leading to a reduction in the number and degree of deformities in new cases and a greater compliance with treatment by patients. In 1991, Member States adopted a resolution in the World Health Assembly (WHA44.9) to eliminate leprosy as a public health problem by the year 2000, that is, to reduce the prevalence to a level below one case per 10 000 population of a country.

Drug abuse. In most cities of the world, problems relating to drug and alcohol abuse and violence have a significant impact on health and place substantial burdens on first-, second-, and third-level health care services. This can be particularly devastating in developing countries where urban health services also have to deal with illness caused by lack of clean water and sanitation, immunization, and basic care.

Mental impairment. Despite the great gains in knowledge made in previous decades in relation to the prevention of mental and neurological disorders and their treatment, particularly in terms of new drugs and new types of psychosocial interventions, a great proportion of people with such disorders do not benefit from these advances. There are also great inequalities in service provision and availability among and within countries and different population segments; the underprivileged – women, children, the elderly, unemployed persons, the homeless, refugees, migrants – bear the heaviest share of disorders and have the least access to care.

Blindness. The technology for simple inexpensive surgery for cataracts exists and such surgery is performed in many developing countries by primary health care workers. However, in many of them, especially in remote areas, equipment and properly trained personnel are not available. As a result, approximately 13 million blind people in developing countries still need cataract surgery. Trachoma and other communicable eye diseases are gradually being brought under control in many countries, but remain a serious problem, especially in less developed rural areas and urban slums, where sanitation is poor. Ocular onchocerciasis and xerophthalmia remain problems, despite the existence of inexpensive and effective technologies for prevention and control – *Simulium* control and ivermectin for onchocerciasis, and vitamin A supplements and nutrition education for vitamin A deficiency blindness.

Tuberculosis. National tuberculosis programmes are not functioning satisfactorily in many countries in the developing world; it is estimated that fewer than half of existing tuberculosis cases are detected and fewer than half of those detected are cured. However, a number of countries have shown that tuberculosis programmes can achieve, on a countrywide scale and under a variety of conditions, at least an 80% cure rate when short-course chemotherapy is combined with strong programme management. Furthermore, evaluation of these programmes has shown that well-managed tuberculosis control is one of the most cost-effective health interventions available.

Chronic diseases. Many developing countries are already in, or are soon to enter, a period of marked demographic and epidemiological transition, and their health services will have added responsibilities for prevention and care of many diseases including cancer and the provision of related pain relief, chronic cardiovascular diseases, and many other chronic diseases including diabetes mellitus and arthritis.

Radiotherapy and radiology. Although radiotherapy and nuclear medicine facilities do exist in many developing countries, approximately 70% of people still do not have access to the most basic X-ray diagnostic services. Facilities that do exist are often concentrated in the capital cities and other big urban areas, and 30–60% of equipment is estimated not to function. The basic radiographic system is relatively inexpensive and as effective a diagnostic and therapeutic tool as much more costly equipment, but only 700–800 of these units are installed worldwide. It is a paradox that a system conceived for the developing world has proved to be the equipment of choice in developed countries with ample resources, where value for money is the criterion, and is much less used in developing countries. The purchase of a more expensive machine when equally effective equipment – which is easier to run and maintain – is available is an unnecessary waste of scarce technical and financial resources and contributes to care being of poorer quality than it should be.

Resources. The demands placed on health systems and services may have to be met with lower levels of financial, human, and technical resources than were previously available. The quantity and quality of some, or all, elements of health care may inevitably decline. One of the least reported aspects of health development is the status of quality of care. However, there are clues from the increasing number of evaluations of specific aspects of primary health care, predominantly in the areas of immunization, diarrhoeal disease control, and maternal and child health care and family planning. There is some evidence to suggest that in areas supported with extensive technology, coverage can be increased while maintaining quality. When the infrastructure (i.e., staff and facilities) is expanded without expanding the necessary support (drugs and supplies, vehicles, logistics, maintenance,

and resources for supervision), quality of care has declined.

Laboratory services. The availability of efficient and reliable laboratory services is an essential element of care – to diagnose anaemia, malaria, tuberculosis, and other infectious and parasitic diseases; to help in decisions about treatment; to check that therapy has worked; to test blood for transfusion. A misdiagnosis of a disease made on the basis of a laboratory test can have devastating consequences for an individual, his family or his community. For example, the impact on someone who does not have AIDS but believes that he or she does because of a false laboratory test is unimaginable. Furthermore, such false positive results can have serious financial and technical repercussions for the health care system itself. It can equally be a problem when a laboratory test wrongly indicates no infection (a false negative result). For example, streptococcal infection can be safely and inexpensively treated with antibiotics and does not require referral to second- or third-level care. In contrast an untreated infection may lead to the much more serious and costly condition of rheumatic heart disease. In developing countries rheumatic fever and rheumatic heart disease account for more than three out of ten cardiac cases admitted to hospital – a needless waste of technical and financial resources and a needless cause of human suffering.

Increasingly, in many developing countries, efficient and reliable laboratory services are becoming available at the local level. Some countries, however, still overemphasize the development of central laboratories to support second- and third-level care, and this in turn often leads to delays in treatment for those in need at more peripheral levels. The chronic shortage of funds in many developing countries has made the extension of laboratory services at peripheral level difficult in some cases. Shortages of funds also lead to supplies of poor quality (hence unreliable) reagents. Additional problems include poor selection and unsatisfactory installation of equipment or poor maintenance leading to equipment breakdown; weak or non-existent quality assurance activities; and shortages of adequately trained staff.

Blood transfusion. Blood transfusion services have been improved in many countries, largely because AIDS has focused attention on the need to improve the safety of blood and blood products. Specific action to develop a safe blood supply and rationalize the use of blood is under way in 149 countries. Strategies are aimed at ensuring safety at source (through the recruitment of voluntary blood donors), excluding infected blood through screening, improving laboratory and manufacturing practices and quality control. Comparing 1986 data with early 1991, there has been an increase in the number of countries screening blood for HIV, and great strides have been made in rationalizing blood transfusion practices – as in Uganda and Zaire, where the prescribing of blood transfusion has been drastically reduced.

AIDS. AIDS alone has placed great additional burdens on the already strained health sector in many developing countries. In the developing world the overall social and economic impact of the pandemic will be immense and the health and social support infrastructure will be inadequate to handle the clinical burden of HIV-related disease. Through the deaths of millions of young men and women, the elderly will be left without support, and 10 million children in sub-Saharan Africa alone will be orphaned by the year 2000, all of which will add further strain to the health and social sectors.

Most Member States have national AIDS programmes and, as of 31 December 1991, 139 countries were receiving WHO support for their implementation. Progressively, national AIDS control activities have begun to move beyond their initial focus in cities and towns, although resources to implement decentralization are sometimes scarce. Home care and other services available to HIV-infected persons and their families have been analysed in six Latin American and African countries. The lessons learned with regard to innovative ways of planning and implementing effective care outside institutions at a much lower cost will be applicable to many other countries and to health problems other than AIDS.

The paramount need in HIV/AIDS prevention is for information, education, and communication. Many health promotion and education activities are targeted at specific risk groups such as prostitutes, intravenous drug users, and young people through various approaches, including peer outreach activities. In most countries, AIDS information and education activities have been introduced into schools, as part of science and family education. For out-of-school youth, the strategy has been to mobilize Scout groups, youth clubs, and similar associations in the public and private sectors. Health education units in many countries have been significantly strengthened during the past several years. In practically all countries there are advisory committees on information, education, and communication, and they are multisectoral in composition. Communication has been improved through the use of circulars and newsletters and innovative approaches to the design of other printed materials. In virtually all countries with a national AIDS programme, NGOs are very active, predominantly at village level.

Communications. People in remote areas, including those who live in mountainous terrain and on islands, often have more difficult access to care or suffer the consequences of lack of personnel; such simple logistic problems as lack of petrol or out-of-action vehicles affect the availability of supplies or equipment and access to second- or third-level referral services. Even the simple lack of telephone facilities could mean that although referral may not be necessary, advice or guidance cannot be obtained. It is difficult to get personnel to work in remote areas. Often specific population groups have less access to the care and services than they need, be they women and children who have a low status in society, or people who are politically weak such as refugees, street and slum dwellers, victims of war and natural disaster, or the elderly – although, particularly in developed countries, this latter group of people has increasing political influence. Many countries have increased the numbers of health facilities, with special emphasis on rural areas, or have placed a health centre on each atoll or island in island countries. Other countries, including developed countries, use mobile health services to ensure access to basic care and to specialized care for remote populations.

The elderly. Cross-national studies on the needs of the elderly in developing countries from three continents have consistently shown that their main problem is lack of financial resources which in turn prevents large numbers of people from satisfying many of their basic needs and limits their access to health care. Most countries have emphasized the integration of health services for the elderly into other kinds of first-level care. They also emphasize the importance of the informal support system provided by families and the community. Similar importance is attached to this approach for other issues also. For example, maternity benefits, children's day care, home helps, and family allowances are among the approaches adopted by some countries to support families and communities in leading healthier and happier lives. For instance, Israel passed a nursing insurance law in 1986 that allowed the integration of long-term care for the elderly into the community and family by subsidizing personal and home-making services for elderly people. Other countries such as Uruguay have followed suit. But there is another side to such approaches. For example, Scandinavian countries that adopted compensation for ill and disabled patients several years ago, when they were economically prosperous, are now finding that they cannot easily afford them.

Self-care. The right and ability of people to undertake health actions themselves continue to be only partially recognized. Yet people do provide a great deal of care for themselves, their families, and their communities, without any contact with formal health care or services; most of this care is provided by women, in their capacity as mothers and principal care-givers in their families or in their important – albeit often unacknowledged – roles as motivators and principal supports of many different (social, health, and developmental) activities in their communities. Increasingly, too, people demand to be involved in, and responsible for, more of their health care. Often the involvement of people and communities is a pragmatic necessity; without their involvement in health promotion, disease prevention, and the care of the sick and of people with disabilities, some people would have little or no care and much "formal" health care would have a limited or short-term impact. Individuals and communities have always assumed much responsibility – for example, in caring for the elderly, the chronically ill, people with disabilities, people with AIDS, and psychiatric patients who have been "de-institutionalized", and this burden of responsibility may be increasing. This increase is the result not simply of the inability of the health sector to provide the necessary care, for technical or for financial reasons, but of the desire of individuals and communities to provide this care because they feel that institutional care is not appropriate to what people need or is lacking in compassion.

Nongovernmental organizations. The role of nongovernmental organizations in health care is significant in many countries where resources are scarce. They are also very important in linking the community with the health sector, with other sectors, and to local governments. Nongovernmental organizations have continued to play a crucial role in providing expertise and resources, especially at community level. Their awareness of local cultural and religious sensitivities, for example, makes them especially effective partners in working with individuals and communities. In addition to their financial, technical and managerial skills and resources, they are often instrumental in the training of health personnel and in community education and mobilization. Although voluntary organizations are nationally organized in a number of countries, the lack of a policy framework for coordinating their efforts remains a significant obstacle to the full utilization of their skills and resources.

In turn, these trends and developments have many implications for the responsibility and roles of health services. Health workers have had to improve their working relationships with each other and with other sectors, and to learn to work with people rather than just providing services to them. The training of health personnel has begun to change in some cases. Many institutions in both developing and developed countries are now using innovative new approaches to education and training such as community-oriented training and problem-based curricula for health personnel at all levels. It must be borne in mind, however, that whether they are educated in innovative ways or according to more traditional methods, health personnel cannot efficiently and effectively undertake the tasks for which they have been trained when equipment and supplies are lacking or of poor quality, when logistics systems fail, or when the health systems in which they must work are not fully functional. In addition to the demoralization and demotivation that this can lead to, it is a waste of very valuable human resources.

Health promotion. Health promotion is social and political action at individual and collective levels aimed at enhancing public awareness of health, at fostering healthy life styles and at creating conditions conducive to health. It is a process of activating communities, policy-makers, professionals, and the public for sustained behavioural change (reducing behaviour that is risky to health and adopting health-enhancing behaviour) and for bringing about the environmental changes that would reduce or eliminate social and other environmental causes of ill health. The developed countries have put particular emphasis on promoting healthy life styles to minimize the risk of diseases and on creating supportive environments for health. In developing countries, particular stress is placed on enlisting active community involvement in ensuring basic sanitation and water supply, maternal and child care, and the control of communicable diseases. Obviously much common ground is shared by the primary health care approach and the concept of health promotion (7).

Health education. Increasingly, health education for individuals and communities is aimed at providing the various kinds of knowledge and skills that lay people need in view of their increasing interest and responsibilities in health, so that they can act individually and collectively to help to shape services and care rather than to be merely the passive recipients of professional services and decisions made by other people. Training of trainers is an essential strategy, in order to obtain a multiplier effect both for education and training for health personnel and for lay people. Many countries have strengthened their health education units and increasingly information and education activities in schools and specific activities focus on youth groups, associations and clubs for out-of-school youth. There also is increased emphasis on the use of the media to reach individuals and population groups in both developed and developing countries as well as awareness of the influence that the mass media have on health – for example, advertising bias.

Conclusion

Indicator 7 comprises four elements of care, each of which in turn comprises a number of subelements of care. Countries have not provided information on the extent of coverage with *all* of these elements or subelements. Therefore, these data can only give an approximation of trends in comprehensive coverage. These problems notwithstanding, the data do show that coverage with the individual elements of primary health care identified by global indicator 7 is increasing globally. It must be borne in mind, however, that some of these individual elements of indicator 7 ask for information about two or more issues; for example, one element asks about "safe water in the home or within reasonable access *and* with adequate excreta-disposal facilities available". Countries have given information about coverage with safe water (i.e., Fig. 3.1) and about coverage with excreta-disposal facilities (i.e., Fig. 3.2), but not about coverage with both of these complementary subelements of care. Similarly, information has been provided by countries for coverage with the different immunizations included in the indicator – but not for all vaccinations. The same problem is seen with separate information on coverage with care for mothers during pregnancy and during deliveries and for care of children.

Differences in coverage continue to exist between countries, and there is evidence that in a number of cases the differences between developed countries and those characterized as least developed is increasing. By implication, differences between groups within countries may also be on the rise.

The reasons for these differences are well known; many of them have been referred to in this chapter. In part, the problems and solutions lie within the health sector itself, where health care is often provided through vertical programmes. These give visibility to individual diseases and health problems and may be the most effective way to deal with certain problems. However, the provision of vertical programmes can encourage fragmented approaches to care. It may not take sufficient account either of the total range of action needed in the health sector and outside it, by health personnel and by individuals in the private and public sectors. Furthermore, it tends to accentuate the curative and rehabilitative elements of health care to the detriment of disease prevention and health maintenance; it focuses on disease and problems rather than on people and does not take adequate account of the contribution that people themselves make to maintaining their health and to caring for and curing illness. Integration means different things to different systems, but generally involves the expansion of case-finding and treatment tasks performed by multipurpose facilities and staff. Appropriate degrees of integration must be determined within each country's system, and this can take time.

The source of some of the problems and many of the answers are also to be found outside the health sector: in the overall value system of societies, including the commitment of governments to maintaining and improving the health of peoples through the variety of appropriate means and their commitment to ensuring literacy and education, in political, economic, and demographic factors, in development policies, in technological and scientific developments, and in the policies and orientations of external aid agencies.

Better coordination between policy-makers in different sectors and better coordination between complementary programmes that impact on health implemented in those sectors is also essential if conflicts of interest are to be avoided, just as better coordination of efforts within the health sector is needed in order to prevent the duplication of effort, to ensure that the most efficient use is made of human and financial resources and to maximize opportunities to improve health. To cite but one example of the impact of improved coordination in the health sector alone: if one health service vaccinates infants – who are usually brought by their mothers – the same service could also vaccinate the mothers against tetanus, thereby enabling the coverage of women of child-bearing age with tetanus toxoid to approach the levels of vaccination coverage of infants and children.

Objectives and programme targets, be they at national or health sector level, are similarly often expressed in terms of specific services to be provided or of reducing specific diseases instead of identifying goals. In some ways this is a reflection of the training of health personnel, policy-makers, economists, and funding agencies. In other respects, it is a reflection of the durability of attitudes and practices and familiar ways of doing things. It is also a reflection of the way in which resources are allocated. However, it is becoming increasingly evident that health is the result of action – or inaction – in many sectors. This has implications for the ways in which the various sectors must learn to think about and work with each other.

Fig. 3.9 shows the various partners in health development, i.e., the public and private sectors, nongovernmental organizations, the community and the family, as well as bilateral and multilateral agencies. The district health care services are the basic infrastructure for the delivery of integrated health care, and it is at this level of the system that the common approach to solving interrelated health problems should be emphasized. If the various disease problems are considered in isolation, and funded accordingly, the effectiveness of scarce resources cannot be optimized – all the components of the system should function in a coordinated and integrated manner if the health sector is to be efficient and effective in improving the health of the individual. District health services should also draw more extensively on the potential energy of families and communities, in order to make better use of resources that will remain limited, and may even diminish further. However the value system associated with development, the environment and life styles will determine how close the district health system and services available in the community can be brought together, and how much can be achieved. If full use were

Fig. 3.9
Partners in health development

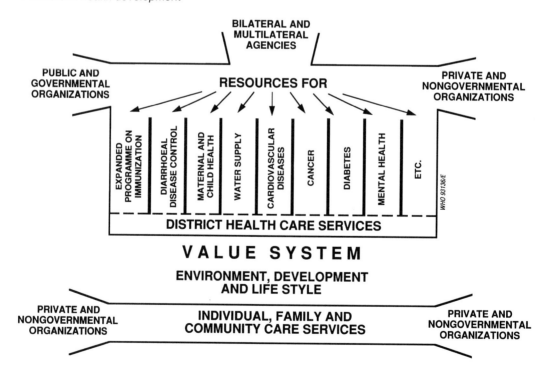

made of the complementarity and potential for mutual reinforcement of the various partners, and if essential care covering all eight elements of primary health care were provided on an integrated basis, present achievements in improving health service coverage could be maintained and inequities in health status could be reduced.

References

1. *Global strategy for health for all by the year 2000.* Geneva, World Health Organization, 1981 ("Health for All" Series, No. 3).

2. *World conference on education for all: meeting basic learning needs, Jomtien, Thailand, 5–9 March 1990. Final report.* New York, Inter-Agency Commission (UNDP, UNESCO, UNICEF, World Bank) for the World Conference on Education for All, 1990.

3. *Barrier methods.* Baltimore, MD, Johns Hopkins University Population Information Program, 1990 (Population reports, Series H, No. 8)

4. *Safe motherhood: a tabulation of available data on the frequency and mortality of unsafe abortion.* Geneva, World Health Organization, 1990 (document WHO/MCH/90.14).

5. *Hospitals and health for all.* Geneva, World Health Organization, 1987 (Technical Report Series, No. 744: report of a WHO Expert Committee on the role of hospitals at the first referral level).

6. *Case-mix management experiences in European countries: options and opportunities for the acute hospital sector.* Paris, Organisation for Economic Co-operation and Development, 1991 [document SME/ELSA/WP1(91)20].

7. *Health promotion in developing countries.* Geneva, World Health Organization, 1991 (briefing book to the Sundsvall conference on supportive environments, 1991: document WHO/HED/91.1).

CHAPTER 4

Health resources

Introduction

Resource patterns summarize past commitments to health and provide concrete evidence of successes and failures in meeting policy objectives. This review of global trends in health resources from 1985 to 1990 begins with a consideration of changes in the overall level of financial resources for health, from both governments and nongovernmental sources, and outlines recent policy trends in the financing and organization of the health care system and in the deployment of human resources and the development of technologies for health.

Several different approaches are commonly used in measuring the level of financial resources available for health. The percentage of government expenditure devoted to health allows an assessment of the relative priority given to health by comparison with other government expenditure commitments, such as education, defence, and economic services. Data from the International Monetary Fund (*1*), which are limited to central government expenditures, show that for the period since 1985 for which data are available, health as a percentage of government spending increased globally, although there were regional variations.

However, the size of the government sector in the overall economy is itself subject to change. A constant share of government expenditure on health could be a constant, growing, or diminishing amount of total national income. Global indicator 3 thus measures the percentage of GNP spent on health, based on central government expenditures (see Fig. 4.1 and box). The most striking feature of the data shown here is the difference in share of GNP allocated to health between the developed and the developing countries. These data are broadly consistent with the trends reported by the IMF (*1*).

National income levels, however, are also liable to fluctuate, particularly in developing countries, when the combined effects of inflation and population growth are taken into account. A recent World Bank report states: "Nearly one half of a sample of 90 nations monitored closely by the Bank experienced falling real income per capita ... in the 1980s. Only a dozen or so developing countries experienced a significant increase in per capita income" (*2*). Perhaps the most instructive indicator of trends in resources for health is thus real per capita health spending, which shows whether the health resources available to each individual are growing, shrinking, or remaining constant over time. Data show that, for major developed countries, real per capita health spending increased in the period since 1985. For middle-income and less developed countries the picture is much more variable. A 1990 World Bank study indicated that, for a sample of 20 African countries, real health spending was higher in 1987 than in 1980 (*3*). However, these conclusions appear to be sensitive to the method of calculation employed, and the same data actually show a substantial decline when the averages are

Global indicator 3

The percentage of gross national product spent on health

Fig. 4.1

Percentage of GNP spent on health by central government (global indicator 3), 1985 and 1991

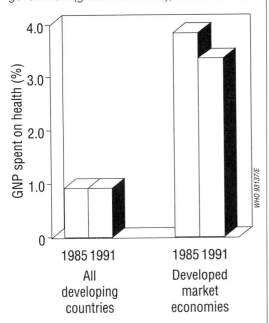

weighted by population size. It is clear that experiences vary widely on this criterion of health resources and that more detailed analysis is required.

All the above indicators are based on data for spending by central government. They thus omit not only health expenditures by other levels of government, but all resources contributed by the nongovernment sector. In some countries, state or provincial expenditures for health are an important share of the total (India, Nigeria, USA), and may have become increasingly so in the period since 1985. In all countries, the nongovernment health sector is an important, and often growing, part of health finance and provision (see Fig. 4.2). Thus the available data tend to understate, in an increasingly unsystematic fashion, the current picture of resource availability for health.

Financial resources for health

The value of government health expenditures on citizens in most developed countries is often greater than total per capita income in the least developed countries. For example, per capita health spending in western Europe in 1987 averaged just under US$ 900 (*4*), between three and four times the total per capita income of Uganda, Mali or Myanmar. Health financing and overall economic development are related. Broadly speaking, the richer the country, the higher the proportion of its income it allocates for health, as shown in Fig. 4.3.

There are important exceptions to the general trend of increasing health expenditure with income levels, however, as the ranges surrounding these averages show. Some countries spend substantially more on health than the average for their level of income and others substantially less. Examples include Botswana, Papua New Guinea, and Sri Lanka, which spend more than their per capita income group average, and Bangladesh and Uganda, which spend less.[1]

In general, richer countries spend more on health, though greater spending is not always associated with better health outcomes. The continued effects of environment, life style and biology are more influential in determining health status than are health services in isolation.

A country with a lower income than another, and with lower health expenditure, may still have better health. For example, Sierra Leone

---

1. These data refer only to central government expenditures for health. They are therefore incomplete, as they omit expenditures by local or state governments (in countries such as Nigeria and India these are major parts of public sector spending for health). In addition these data do not reflect nongovernment health expenditures, which are often greater than government spending.

Fig. 4.2

Private expenditure on health as a percentage of total health expenditure, around 1987

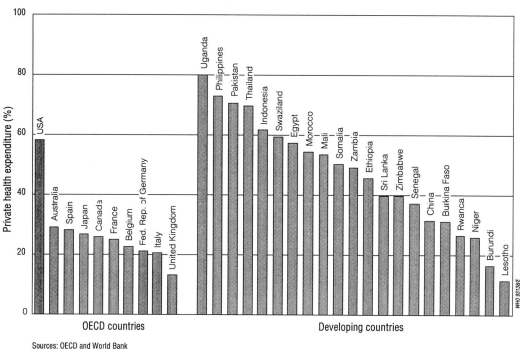

Sources: OECD and World Bank

and Sri Lanka both have incomes of about US$ 400 per annum. But Sri Lanka's life expectancy at birth is over 70 years, while that of Sierra Leone is less than 50. Peru and Costa Rica both have per capita incomes of about US$ 1500, but life expectancy at birth in Costa Rica is over 10 years greater than in Peru, and infant mortality patterns in these countries show similar divergences. In fact, Costa Rica's life expectancy at birth and infant mortality are as good as those of the Federal Republic of Germany, though its per capita income is less than one tenth of the Federal Republic's. The effectiveness of social policy relates as much to the way in which resources are distributed and the populations to whom they are available as it does to the total value of the resources used.

International differences in economic growth and demographic trends, referred to in chapter 1, have contributed to a variety of experiences with government expenditure. Real per capita GNP has fallen since 1985 in many developing countries, while it has grown in most developed market economies. Even when governments have maintained the share of public resources committed to health, as in Ghana or Papua New Guinea and as discussed in chapter 1, this may have meant a fall in real per capita health spending. In many more cases, stagnant or declining national income has been accompanied by retrenchment in public spending which has reduced the share of health in government spending since 1985 (China, Philippines).

Whatever the trends in national economic growth and the share of national income allocated to health by government, it is clear that, for most developing countries, the combined effects of inflation and population growth have

Fig. 4.3
Government health expenditure as a percentage of GNP, 1987

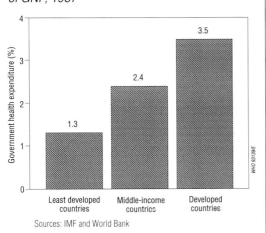

Sources: IMF and World Bank

resulted in declining real public spending for health per capita. Thus, recent data for Ghana (Fig. 4.4), where the share of health in government spending has increased between 1985 and 1990, show that, adjusting for inflation and population growth, 1990 health spending was around US$ 6 per person – about the same level as in 1986 or 1980, but substantially less than in 1978, the year of the Alma-Ata Declaration. The United Republic of Tanzania also reports that 1988–1989 expenditure figures for health were 10% lower in real per capita terms than in 1980–1981. In addition to this absolute decline in government spending experienced in a number of countries, there has been a relative fall in government versus nongovernment spending in many more. For many developing countries, particularly in Africa, economic reality in health has been one of shrinking government capability. Several studies have established that the poor are more dependent on publicly provided health services than the rich. A declining share of health financing by government constitutes an important potential threat to equitable access to health care and an early warning of widening differences in health status

among richer and poorer populations within a country.

The developed countries, on the other hand, have continued to increase their real health spending per capita. A recent OECD study (4) reports an average real health expenditure growth for Canada, France, Federal Republic of Germany, Italy, Japan, the United Kingdom and the United States of 3.3% per annum for the period 1975–1987, with an average population growth of only 0.5%.

Reports from WHO regions reflect this diversity of experience. In Africa up to 90% of the total public funding for health in a small number of countries, and 20% in several more, is now from external sources. Per capita health spending is under US$ 5 per annum in about one-quarter of the countries in Africa. Similar figures are reported for Bangladesh, Pakistan, and India. Countries with higher average per capita income also recognized resource constraints as a major limitation on their health system development but, in addition, acknowledged ineffective use and inadequate information on expenditure and costs as contributory elements in the overall resource problem. All countries in WHO's South-East Asia Region reported concern about resource constraints, and expressed special concern about inequities in their distribution. Economic performance varies substantially among countries in the region, from Thailand's average growth of nearly 9% per annum, 1985–1990, to Myanmar's negative growth, 1985–1989.

In the WHO Western Pacific Region, which has experienced political stability and an average economic growth rate of 6% in 1989 and 1990, and where expected growth over the remainder of the 1990s is 2–3% per annum, recovery from the recession of the early 1980s was relatively rapid. Concern with the level of resources in this region, as in other higher-income regions, is reported to relate less to questions of mobilization than to questions of utilization. These countries concur that the greatest extra

Fig. 4.4

Real expenditure on health per capita, Ghana, 1978–1990

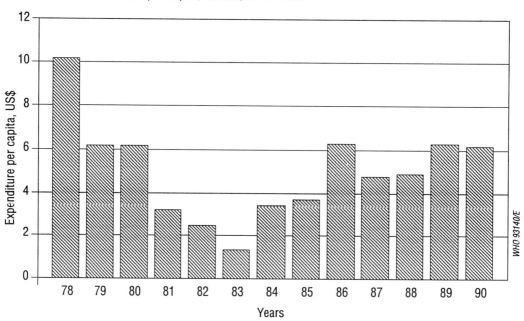

value in financial terms is likely to come through improved efficiency in coordination, management, and utilization. Quality assurance, improved and decentralized budgeting arrangements, and the use of cost-effectiveness criteria were reported as ways of pursuing these efficiency savings (China).

Several countries report the development of recent financial master plans for health (e.g., Papua New Guinea), but there is a common lack of information about the activities of the nongovernment health sector and the nature of its interaction with the public sector. The majority of developing countries still do not have a clear overall picture of health financing. For example, the relative size of spending on government services, modern private sector services, mission or other not-for-profit services, community financed activities, and traditional care is often unknown.

Ministries have thus been unable to develop constructive policies to coordinate private and public activities in health. In New Zealand and the Republic of Korea, for example, concern was expressed about the duplication of services as a result of poor coordination between the private and public sectors. In most developing countries, information about the scope of the private sector continues to be provided by periodic household expenditure surveys. The small amount of information available from these suggests that the relative size of the nongovernment sector to the government sector is greater in poorer countries than in middle-income or developed countries, as Fig. 4.2 illustrates.

International aid for health (as mentioned in global indicator 6, see box) is also often recorded incompletely, and relevant information is not available so far. In some countries it is impossible to separate health from population finances. In many more, donors' support is recorded in ways that do not facilitate comparisons with Ministry of Health expenditure.

Global indicator 6
The amount of international aid received or given for health

Growth of the nongovernment sector

Important changes in government policy in the health sector are reported by many countries. In some cases a reorientation in government policy precedes and sets the tone for change in individual sectors. Thus, as part of a general policy of restoring market mechanisms and reducing the direct responsibility of government, Chile has achieved a major shift in the financing pattern of its health care in the past decade, moving from a centrally funded, tax-based system through a social-security-based system to one that now relies substantially on private funding supported by both compulsory and voluntary insurance schemes.

In Czechoslovakia, the restructuring of the health sector is being undertaken as a leading component in the development of a pluralistic social and economic structure, in a deliberate attempt to democratize and move away from a monolithic, top-down, government bureaucracy.

In addition to Czechoslovakia, all of the other former centrally planned economies in central and eastern Europe began planning conspicuous changes in the role of government. The general shape of new health systems in Albania, Bulgaria, Hungary, Poland, Romania, and the USSR is not yet clear. Social and political changes are being implemented at a time of profound economic crisis, so the full effects of this restructuring will not appear for several years. Each country's system is likely to differ from its neighbour's, but all are being designed to improve the quality, equity, and accountability of health care. Much of the current debate centres on steps in the transition process to a social-insurance-based system, but urgent short-term problems such as the pay of health workers and the right to undertake private practice are being faced.

In Namibia, independence in 1990 cleared the way for a major shift in the role of government. That country has now begun to abolish an inequitable and fragmented set of health care systems based on race, and to develop a system geared to meeting the health needs of all its population, based on a primary health care approach. Substantial progress in the development of district-based health systems and of community financing initiatives is reported in a majority of countries in Africa. Similar movements away from central government control of financing and provision of health services are being pursued at differing paces in numerous other countries, at all levels of development.

In some countries, governments have been forced into making policy changes as a result of rapidly changing economic circumstances. In Nigeria, for example, a recent rapid deterioration in the economy resulted in a sharp decline in the quality of care available from government sources. A surge in private sector activity is now creating growing inequities, and is compelling governments to reconsider both how to manage the relationship between the public and private sectors, and how to restore competitiveness in the public sector. Several countries report a rapid growth in the private sector. Thailand reports that almost 80% of its health expenditure is now from private household payments. In Cyprus the total share of health (public and private) in GNP has grown slowly since 1985 from 3.9% to 4.2% in 1989, but the private sector component has grown rapidly and currently accounts for over 60% of this share. A recent study in India also estimates household payments at 60% of total health expenditure. In Iran, about 35% of health expenditures are for nongovernment services.

Trends in the public/private mix in health resources

Many governments, recognizing their incapacity to finance and administer comprehensive health services for whole populations, are viewing nongovernmental agencies with new interest. In the 1970s and much of the 1980s, the roles of the private sector and other nongovernmental agencies such as missions or parastatal agencies in health were relatively neglected. The main sources of attention, outside the public sector, were traditional practitioners and community-based health initiatives. Some countries report successful experiences in linkages with these important elements of the health system (e.g., China, the Democratic People's Republic of Korea, Viet Nam). In other countries, however, effective coordination by government has often proved difficult, and regulation by government has sometimes been counterproductive, particularly when government financial regulations conflict with the way in which communities wish to manage their resources.

Falling real wages in the public sector, increasing costs of imported goods such as pharmaceuticals, vehicles, fuel and medical equipment, and a growing dependence on cost-sharing by external donors and users of health services have pressed many governments to review their role and relationships with nongovernmental health agencies. In addition, the economic impact of AIDS on the health system has been substantial in both rich and poor countries. In rich countries AIDS raises health care costs. In poorer countries, where resources already do not match needs, the treatment of patients with AIDS tends to divert funds from services for patients with other ailments.

Two broad areas of innovation have been tried in countries at all levels of development with: (1) changes in the pattern of financing; and (2) changes in arrangements for service provision. In undertaking these changes, the regulatory approaches and mechanisms used by governmental and other agencies have also changed substantially.

Changes in the pattern of financing

A major change in financing in both rich and poor countries has often occurred without direct government policy encouragement: reliance on out-of-pocket payments for privately provided services. As explained above, this has been seen in many countries in the form of a rapid growth in private practice at a time when the utilization of many government health facilities is falling. Many pre-existing government regulations about private practice have proved unenforceable.

Governments have also initiated financing changes by policies towards health insurance. Thus, Indonesia and Sri Lanka have taken measures to promote voluntary health insurance; Malaysia is exploring ways to encourage private health insurance in rural areas. Many more countries are appraising the feasibility of extending or introducing compulsory health insurance systems. The Republic of Korea has now extended its compulsory insurance system to provide near-total coverage. Like many health systems financed by insurance, it is now facing cost escalation.

New or increased levels of fees for health services provided by government have perhaps been more widely used than any other single policy vehicle for increasing health finances. The only important group of countries that appears to be an exception to this trend is the developed countries, where co-payment levels appear to have stabilized in the past five years at between 10–20% of total costs. User fees can be a politically difficult issue at times of economic crisis, as experience in Kenya showed, since they limit access by the poor but often contribute little or nothing to total revenues because of low yields and administrative leakages. Some developing countries have found that increases in fees, without accompanying changes in the quality of services, simply divert needy and poorer patients to other sources of care (e.g., Lesotho, Swaziland) and decrease utilization at government facilities. Differentiated fee systems, which are administratively more complex, operate in Mexico and Zimbabwe, based on patients' income levels. As in other types of fee system, the level of charges needs to be modified periodically to keep up with inflation.

The technical discussions at the 1987 World Health Assembly addressed the question of economic support for Health for All and set out key criteria for the assessment of any potential change in financing mechanisms.

Many nongovernmental agencies appear to be more successful than their government counterparts in recovering costs through fees and in using the revenues to improve services. Religious missions, for example, often appear to combine substantial cost recovery, good quality of care, and access for the genuinely poor. This suggests that well-run cost-recovery schemes, like well-run health services, depend fundamentally on motivated and capable managers. There is, however, a widespread acceptance among populations of the need to pay for certain health goods, such as pharmaceuticals. Cost-recovery schemes, usually local in scale and based on essential drugs, have been successful in several countries (Benin, Guinea-Bissau, the Lao People's Democratic Republic). Community financing initiatives, such as those encouraged by the Bamako initiative, are often more than a mechanism for mobilizing additional funding for health. They frequently involve wider participation in management of the scheme and thus encompass changes in both financing and provision of services.

Some countries now have experience with private health provision in public facilities, which in some cases may be a means of generating additional finance for the public sector, as when beds are leased to the private sector. Several countries in the African region report new or planned arrangements for intramural private practice. However, there are also many in-

Ghana

Raising fees for government health services (5)

The Ghanaian economy faced many problems in the early 1980s: population growth exceeded growth in food production, and inflation was over 100%. Per capita income fell by one-third between 1974 and 1982. Economic problems, compounded by rising debt repayments, led Ghana to introduce an IMF-supported recovery programme in 1983. Fees for health care were increased in 1983 and again, more substantially, in 1985.

In the urban health facilities of one region, outpatient utilization halved following the 1985 fee increase. Over subsequent years urban utilization levels gradually increased to the pre-1985 level. But in rural areas utilization fell even further, and had still not recovered to 1985 levels five years later, in spite of continuing rapid population growth. The age composition of users of government health services also changed, with an increase in use by those in the 15–45 age group, and a decline in other groups, most strongly among those aged over 45. Similar trends were reported for the country as a whole. The cost-recovery target (15% of recurrent costs) was achieved in the immediate post-increase period, although it has not been sustained since, as costs have increased faster than charges. There were long delays in making decisions on how to spend the revenue collected and little evidence of an improvement in service quality. Observers commented that cost recovery had focused too closely on money and not enough on the health consequences of financing changes. Subsequent modifications to the system have included "cash and carry" schemes for purchasing drugs, in which each health unit manages its own budget for pharmaceuticals.

stances of unplanned or unregulated "poaching" of public resources for private practice, creating subsidies at public expense for patients who are relatively well off.

Changes in health care provision

Changes in public and private sector roles in the provision of health care have also become widespread in recent years. One common modality is the contracting out of certain provision responsibilities that had previously been the exclusive concern of the public sector. Many countries, at all levels of development, have experience of contracting out nonclinical services to the private sector. Common contracts for non-clinical services involve laundry, security, cleaning, catering, waste disposal, and equipment maintenance (Malaysia, United Kingdom). In other cases, certain diagnostic services and clinical care responsibilities have also been contracted out. The requirements for successful contracting out include the availability of a local market for the service in question, good management, and tight cost-control by the contract-issuing agency.

Other changes in provision are resulting from a more supportive attitude by the public sector to certain roles for the nongovernment sector. Several countries with relatively high levels of coverage are encouraging the notion that patients should have greater freedom to choose among health providers, as a means of encouraging quality-based competition among general practitioners, health centres or hospitals (Chile, Hungary, France, Sweden). Developing countries that had previously banned private practice are in some cases repealing this legislation (Mozambique, United Republic of Tanzania) or allowing greater scope to nongovernment providers by relaxing regulations on fee levels or actively subsidizing private practice in underserved areas.

Policy measures to restore the competitiveness of the public sector as compared to the private sector are being implemented in countries such as Nigeria, where increased pay to government doctors has attracted private practitioners back to government service; and Iran, where fee-for-service practice in certain hospitals provides additional revenue for the hospital as well as for the health workers.

Changing approaches to regulation

The political orientation of the health system in many countries has been influenced by concern about liberalization, decentralization and privatization. These influences affect the health sector in ways that depend importantly on each country's existing level of development and on the structure of the health care system. A widely shared recent experience, however, has been that regulation by central government control and legislation needs to be confined to a selected set of strategic activities, such as prospective budgeting for total public sector spending on health. It is increasingly recognized that regulation has hitherto tended to be too prescriptive and directive; it has also been inadequately negotiated in cases where it has changed incentive structures.

Regulation is commonly understood to include all the mechanisms that determine the location, quantity, quality and prices of health services. In addition to the important contribution of government, the potential or actual roles of at least three additional agents is increasingly being recognized. These are (1) professional bodies (e.g., in monitoring quality of care), (2) third-party financing agencies, such as social security and health insurance funds, which have substantial influence on provider behaviour, and (3) consumers themselves. Different concerns can be distinguished among countries at different levels of development. Most developed countries already have very high levels of coverage and near-universal access to care through public funding of health services. For example, the 1987 average public share (including social insurance) of hospital in-patient costs in 22 developed countries was estimated at over 96% in an OECD report (*4*), although for the United States the figure was only 55%. Most developed countries are concerned with cost pressures due to the increasing age of their populations, the cost of new technologies and procedures, and continuously increasing expectations. A common recent feature in many developed countries has been the adoption of national or provincial prospective "global budgets" to govern health spending. The allocation of these resources is then determined by professional associations and health funding agencies.

Improvements in health sector performance in developed countries is focused on re-invigorating the public sector, in some cases (Spain, Sweden, United Kingdom) restructuring it to increase the regulatory roles of consumers, funding agencies and health professionals and to reduce the detailed managerial responsibility of central government.

"Managed competition" and "internal markets" are phrases used to describe a variety of mechanisms designed to ensure that the financing and providing roles are separated, that health finances follow the patient, and that providers of care compete for service contracts for population groups. Whilst several countries report such changes, it is still too early to forecast their consequences in terms of service integration, popular acceptance, equity, and health outcomes.

Countries in central and eastern Europe are exploring ways of improving pay, morale, quality and equity in their health sectors through transferring different degrees of financing responsibilities to third-party (insurance) payers and to consumers. Like most developing countries, they are at present in deep economic crisis, and they are thus attempting to engineer long-term strategies while coping with shortages, disillusioned health workers and patients, and widespread under-the-counter payments. Plans for social insurance systems are now detailed in some countries and private practice is recognized. But the new structures and regulatory mechanisms are not yet in place, and the new resources to come from restored economic growth are not yet available.

The developing countries are highly heterogeneous in relation to both health systems and economic circumstances. Those that experienced economic growth during the period to 1990 have managed to increase coverage and improve the quality of services. The Annex table (global indicator 4) gives a summary of the responses on the percentage of national health expenditure devoted to local health services. Although the response rate is low, it is noted that in some countries there have been important redefinitions of responsibilities within the health care sector. Thailand's health sector, increasingly financed from private sources, uses 27% of its public budget for first-level health care and over 50% for the rural areas of the country.

Global indicator 4
The percentage of the national health expenditure devoted to local health services

---

China's policy is to give full play to all actors – central government, local authorities, collectives and individuals. Health expenditure in China stood at 3.1% of GNP in 1988. The country reports growing decentralization and a greater attention given to spending money in the most effective way. Large geographical variations in health resources, reflecting regional imbalances in development, remain a major concern, as in many other developing countries. Substantial geographical variations are also reported by India, where total health spending, including the private sector, was estimated to be 3.2% of GNP in 1986-87. Health insurance in middle-income and poor countries typically covers only a fraction of the population. No systematic reports of insurance coverage are at present available from countries, but India's public insurance system appears to cover approximately 4% of the population, Indonesia's just under 10%, those of Iran and the Philippines about 35%, and Mexico's approximately 50%.

Some developing countries have experienced a *de facto* change in roles and responsibilities in the health sector, with the collapse or near collapse of government services. A typical profile of the government health budget is that up to 80% goes on wages and salaries. Other recurrent costs are financed either by patients (e.g., pharmaceuticals) or often not at all (maintenance of buildings and equipment). Chronic recurrent budget problems have led to falling real wages and the neglect of essential maintenance and non-salary running costs. Quality – even when measured in terms of simple indicators such as out-of-stock periods for essential drugs – has fallen. Capital costs in the public sector are increasingly met from foreign assistance sources. Although salaries take such a big share of recurrent costs, a substantial income gap has developed between earnings in the public and the private sectors. The effect is to attract the most qualified health workers out of the public sector, further depleting the quality and morale of the workforce.

Approaches being taken by countries vary and are often piecemeal. Nigeria has increased pay to health workers and undertaken to review rules on private practice in public facilities. Many countries have recent experiences, both positive and negative, with the contracting out to private suppliers of services previously performed by the public sector. In other circumstances, the rationalization of services is being implemented to reduce wastage through duplication (Namibia – duplication caused by racially separated provision; Bolivia – duplication arising from separate administrations for health and social security). Less commonly, health workers have been made unemployed (Ghana, Lao People's Democratic Republic) in order to allow improvements in pay and conditions for remaining public sector workers within the same global bill.

Several of the least developed countries (Afghanistan, Cambodia, Ethiopia, Mozambique, Somalia, Sudan) are in war or postwar situations, and, like other least developed countries, are heavily dependent on foreign assistance: domestic private and government resources for health are inadequate to meet population needs by any criteria. The OECD cites 16 countries in 1987–1988 in which development assistance is greater than 15% of gross national product (7). All but two of these are in Africa. Where foreign assistance is so important, the government's authority may be eclipsed. Countries dependent on foreign aid face problems with the harmonization of donor activities in coordinated programmes designed to establish a basic network of services. These problems include uncertainty regarding the duration and amount of financing, making it difficult for countries to plan for sustainable community services. Similar considerations apply in different degrees to all aid-recipient countries. The short-term aim in the least developed countries continues to be maximizing the effective use of available resources, the development of managerial capacities and sustainable health systems, and overall economic development.

Many Member States expressed continuing concern with internal health inequalities. Such unevenness in the distribution of health resources is often substantial. Where one or two large urban hospitals, even when they function as national referral centres, dominate public spending patterns, these imbalances are inevitable. Making hospitals self-accounting will do little or nothing to change this. In Mali, 50% of the government budget is spent in an area inhabited by 10% of the population and actually used by even less. Distribution imbalances within countries are even more dramatic when ratios of human resources are examined (see below). Tenfold variations in total per capita health spending by the government between best funded and poorest regions are common. These inequities are in practice much bigger when variations in the availability of private sector resources are reckoned. France and the Nordic countries report the use of private and voluntary organizations in helping to redress inequities. In developed countries increasing concern with inequities was reported, with such groups as the unemployed, immigrants, the elderly, and the young often in disadvantaged positions. Policies gradually to make people, rather than health facilities, the basis of resource allocation, as are reported to be used in Papua New Guinea and several developed countries, are within the power of the ministry of health.

Trends in human resources for health

Most countries have identified human resource development as one of the priorities of the health sector. This is hardly surprising since it takes up about 70% of the recurrent health budget, and in many countries the health sector constitutes the largest single employer.

On the basis of available figures in 1984, worldwide there were over 5 million physicians, 8.5 million nurses and midwives, 447 000 dentists, and over 3.5 million health workers in other categories.

It should be mentioned that statistics on the health workforce are far from satisfactory. Many countries rely on professional registers that are far from current and fail to show those who are at present active. Others are limited only to staff employed by the government. Furthermore, mere numbers provide no information on the performance or productivity of the workforce.

The principal problems have shown a consistency over many years. They are:

(1) imbalances of several types; such as oversupply or shortages, geographical maldistribution, and a less than optimum mix of different professional categories (e.g., physicians and nurses);

(2) low productivity related to poor work conditions, low remuneration, and indifferent career opportunities, which tend to lower morale and performance.

The investment period for training health workers is long. For physicians it could be 10 years from entry to medical school to completion of specialty training. This time lag is an important consideration for all planning. Traditionally, planning methods have been largely normative in approach, when, in fact, the roles and responsibilities of each category of personnel need to be considered in the specific context of where the people in that category actually work. A complex host of factors impinges on the health workforce, which makes planning difficult and outcomes less predictable, but it would be naive to deny the critical influence of vested interests of different professions as well as the phenomenon of professionalization.

Such planning exercises as have been carried out have often not been implemented because the budget was not able to sustain them. In the past three years WHO has advocated the extension of planning to include budgetary implications. This requires planners to look at issues such as opportunity costs and potential substitutions for improving the cost-effectiveness of investment in human resources for health. But new methodologies are required in addition to greater experience in this approach. Unfortunately, the sociocultural imperatives still too often require a physician even when the role is ably performed by a nurse.

The excess of physicians is no longer a problem only of certain developed countries such as Australia and Italy. This phenomenon is now recognized in developing countries such as Bangladesh, India, Mexico, and Pakistan. In some developing countries the problem is often due to the inability of the health budget to employ the required numbers of physicians, but this has been aggravated by the closing of employment opportunities in many developed countries and in the Middle East, in the latter because several countries are setting up medical schools of their own.

Unemployed physicians may also be the basis for the proliferation of schools or departments of public health in the last few years, especially in Europe. As clinical opportunities become scarcer, one career option is to move into the public health field.

On a global basis, the relative shortage of nurses continues although it is particularly pronounced in certain countries such as Bangladesh and Pakistan. The extent of geographical inequity is understated by regional comparisons, but even aggregate comparisons show sharp differences: 1984 figures showed that for 10 000 population there were 56 nurses and midwives in the Americas, but only 3.3 in south-east Asia. Nurses are better educated than at any time in the past and are increasingly called upon for more responsible roles. Unfortunately, nursing is still seen as a woman's profession and suffers the same disadvantages – low status and low salary. When other challenging career options are opening up for women it is not surprising that the nursing profession finds difficulty in recruiting new members and retaining them in active service. The solutions are political and sociocultural rather than technical. The matter was thoroughly discussed at the World Health Assembly in 1989, and changes since then are being monitored.

Over many years medical schools have been blamed for training physicians who are not relevant to the service. The search for relevance in medical education is a continuing one, and currently it seems that the problem-based and community-oriented approach offers the best solution to preparing graduates who can respond to the exigencies of modern medical practice. However, it is also true that not enough attention has been paid to the practice environment and remuneration modalities, which exert an equally important influence on professional behaviour.

The political changes that are taking place in central and eastern Europe have already started to influence the health workforce and its prepa-

ration and work patterns. Additional examples of changes at country level include China's human resource strategy, which has several elements: reforms to develop a three-year family doctor for rural service; upgrading of training of village doctors to assistant doctor level; incentives to encourage work in the countryside and at grass-roots level. In India, in contrast, the decision was made not to open new medical colleges but to increase the number of paramedical institutions and strengthen existing ones. Incentive schemes for work in rural areas have been established and several states pay rural practice allowances. In Iran, and in some Indian states, the director of health services is also responsible for medical education. Thailand reports a controversial decision not to increase the total number of doctors but to increase the number and skills of personnel at health centre level and the number of doctors at district hospitals. From 1988 a rural service requirement has existed for dentists and pharmacists. Improvements in regional equity, measured by manpower to population ratios, are reported: the population per doctor fell by half in the most poorly provided regions between 1981 and 1988.

Trends in research and technology

The contribution of newly developed technology to national health for all strategies remains inadequately assessed in most countries.

Each item of technology can be seen as an investment, which has some potential to improve the productivity of the health system but which requires money, time, and people to operate it. Some technologies have the potential to reduce the need for staff or to lower the costs of services by reducing or avoiding hospital stay. Longer-term savings may result from techniques for screening for early-stage disease, when intervention costs are less than for the advanced condition; cervical cancer is an example. The adoption of new technologies in the government sector should thus be subject to standard investment appraisal methods, such as cost-benefit analysis or cost-effectiveness. Furthermore, governments may wish to regulate the purchasing and use of technologies in the nongovernment sector, where they have important implications for manpower, facilities, and finance in the public sector. In some countries, private overinvestment in health equipment such as hospitals or CAT-scanners has led to pressure on the public sector to finance their operation. Recent studies in the United States show that the rates of utilization of facilities increase with the availability of expensive technology such as laboratories and imaging equipment.

Several countries report the establishment of national research priorities related to major diseases or to organizational factors such as manpower and finance. Few report the development of policies or regulatory procedures regarding the adoption of new technologies in either the public or the private sector.

Typical constraints facing researchers in many developing countries are: intellectual isolation, low salaries, limited promotion, few career paths, restricted research choice, and insufficient training. Their work environment is characterized by lack of access to information, inadequate support staff, institutional instability, and weak infrastructure.

Advances in genetic research, especially the splitting and recombining of DNA molecules, have greatly increased the possible uses of biotechnology for human health. The full scope of these possibilities and their social consequences are still unknown, though a number of ethical issues have already emerged and research indicates that screening may eventually uncover the causes of most debilitating diseases and disorders.

Genetic engineering and other sophisticated techniques make it possible to design biological products with specific features, such as industrial enzymes which last longer, more effective versions of old drugs, and new drugs and vaccines. Mass production of monoclonal anti-bodies through biotechnological means has greatly increased the feasibility of using them in diagnostic tests. Of about 200 types of monoclonal-antibody testing kits available, a significant proportion is now accounted for by tests for acquired immunodeficiency syndrome (AIDS). Genetic manipulation has led to more efficient vaccines for the immunization of children against several diseases.

Technological advances that have a bearing on human reproduction have given rise to much debate in both developed and developing countries, in part reflecting conflicts between religious and secular ethical frameworks. The central effect of these advances has been to broaden the range of choice in human reproduction. Research into contraceptive methods has widened the choices available to family planners. These advances have helped developing countries in the implementation of their more comprehensive population policies.

Other biomedical discoveries such as artificial insemination and *in vitro* fertilization have led to dramatic new ways of intervening in human reproductive processes. These methods impose new social problems, which cannot easily be addressed within traditional ethical and legal frameworks.

Amniocentesis permits the detection of all chromosomal abnormalities in the fetus, as well as serious metabolic disorders and fetal neural tube defects. Other prenatal diagnostic tests include ultrasound scanning, fetoscopy, and fluorescent staining. The findings based on these tests may indicate a need for fetal surgery, another recently developed technique. A by-product of these tests is information about the sex of the fetus which could be put to controversial uses, for example, aborting a fetus simply because it was not of the desired sex.

Important new technologies have been developed in the fight against tropical diseases, and WHO has been particularly active in this field. Clinical trials began in 1991 of arteether and artemether, derivatives of the Chinese

---

Technological change: tuberculosis

Recent progress in the field of tuberculosis includes the following:

(1) **Prevention.** The development of new chemotherapeutic techniques to prevent tuberculosis in persons infected with both *Mycobacterium tuberculosis* and HIV.

(2) **Diagnosis.** Recent advances in immunology and molecular biology are facilitating the development of new diagnostic tools. The polymerase chain reaction technique is one that seems particularly promising because of its sensitivity, specificity, and speed.

(3) **Therapeutics.** Several new classes of drugs have been developed, among which the macrolides and quinolones are particularly important because of their potential for treatment of drug-resistant tuberculosis. The drugs are now being evaluated in preclinical and clinical studies.

---

herbal extract qinghaosu. These drugs clear cerebral malaria faster than quinine. Studies are under way as a step towards registration to allow global use of the derivatives against severe and complicated malaria. Studies in West Africa have given preliminary evidence that home-made bednets, impregnated with a biodegradable insecticide to kill mosquitos, can dramatically reduce child mortality.

In the fight against schistosomiasis, studies in animals have confirmed that praziquantel can be combined with the wide-spectrum anti-helminthic benzimidazoles, offering the prospect of dealing with several helminthic infections at a single treatment.

Ivermectin has been shown conclusively to be an effective microfilaricide against onchocerciasis, reducing eye lesions in Africa, and with potential for transmission blocking in one focus in Latin America (Guatemala). Ivermectin has also emerged as an effective microfilaricide against lymphatic filariasis. The bacterium *Bacillus sphaericus* has been developed as an ecologically safe larvicide against mosquito vectors of lymphatic filariasis in polluted waters in urban areas.

Trypanosomiasis (Chagas' disease) due to *Trypanosoma cruzi* is frequent in some Latin American countries. Fumigant cans, insecticidal paints, and simple vector-detection boxes against the triatomine vectors of the disease have been shown in a pilot project in Argentina to be cheap, effective control techniques, which were welcomed by affected communities. A large multi-country study of these techniques has been launched in Argentina, Bolivia, Chile, Honduras, Paraguay and Uruguay. A socioeconomic study in Venezuela demonstrated that people were prepared to take out, and repay, loans to reconstruct their houses according to a design guide which shows how to make houses resistant to the triatomine vectors of trypanosomiasis due to *Trypanosoma cruzi*.

The elimination of leprosy as a public health problem is now within reach. Ofloxacin has been shown to be highly effective against *Mycobacterium leprae*, and to be well tolerated in combination with standard multi-drug therapy. The prospects of reducing the length of treatment to one month are being assessed. The first results of a 29 000 patient trial of a leprosy vaccine in Venezuela – using whole killed *M. leprae* grown in armadillos – were published in 1991.

In the fight against other communicable diseases, examples of recent important developments include the following:

• A new meningococcal group A and C vaccine has been developed. Protocols for clinical trials of immunogenicity have been approved by national authorities in China and the Gambia. This holds promise of long-lasting immunity – paving the way for inclusion in the Expanded Programme on Immunization.

- Vaccine production on continuous cell lines now ensures large quantities of cheap, safe, and potent human rabies vaccines. The method consists in high-cell-density culture in small fermenters with semicontinuous or continuous antigen extraction. This produces large quantities of rabies vaccine in small production units. An efficacious and safe recombinant rabies vaccine has been developed for the oral immunization of wildlife.

- Persons bitten by rabies-infected animals can now be given a shortened period of vaccine treatment. The new approach dramatically decreases the cost of treatment by reducing the number of injections and/or quantities injected (0.1 ml per dose for intradermal schedules).

- The technology for the production of plasma-derived hepatitis B vaccine has been transferred to China, permitting at least one endemic country to partly satisfy its own needs of the vaccine. The application of genetic engineering techniques to produce hepatitis B vaccine has opened up the possibility of a relatively inexpensive vaccine available in large quantities.

- Several "third-generation" cephalosporins and fluorinated quinolones, which are active against all common types of *Neisseria gonorrhoea* and *Haemophilus ducreyi* were marketed and achieved widespread use, at least in developed countries.

Advanced devices using ultrasound, radiation, lasers and magnetic fields have increased the effectiveness of preventive care and early diagnosis. The emergence of computerized interactive medical diagnostic systems helps doctors to make better diagnoses.

The use of new types of medical equipment has facilitated new kinds of operation on the brain, eye and other vital organs which were not possible 10 or 15 years ago. Genetic screening and other new forms of diagnostic testing – for AIDS, for example – raise several issues of individual and social rights. Perhaps the most vexed question is the priority to be given to the development and use of these techniques in relation to other uses of resources in medicine and public health.

Advances in computer technology have eased the lives of individuals with various types of disability, expanding their employment opportunities as well as social contacts. For example, wheelchairs controlled by microprocessors can help make these persons more mobile.

As the costs of new medical equipment have increased, the technical feasibility of such equipment has not necessarily led to its rapid installation and use.

Important recent clinical technologies related to noncommunicable diseases include:

- the development of patient monitoring and resuscitation equipment and other intensive care unit equipment;
- lithotripsy for kidney and gall stones;
- the use of fibre optics in endoscopy, especially for minimally invasive or non-invasive surgery and day care (endoscopic surgery);
- laser technology in surgery;
- biomaterials for implants;
- the development of disposable materials; and
- home care technology.

These technologies continue to increase the range and magnitude of possible surgical and medical treatment and are likely to reduce hospitalization and expand the scope of general practice and home care.

Besides research and development concerned with specific diseases and health care technologies as described above, there are also various applied research activities aimed at raising the standard of health in poverty-stricken populations, and health systems research and development is being undertaken to provide objective and rational information for the planning, monitoring, and evaluation of implementation.

Summary of trends

In developing countries that have experienced stagnation or economic decline during the past five years, resource questions have been focused on mobilizing external assistance and on nongovernment sources of finance, sometimes to the neglect of issues of coordination and management and the neglect also of overall health objectives such as the protection of the most vulnerable. Government financing and provision have often fallen sharply (Cameroon, Guinea-Bissau, Senegal), (1) so communities have found other ways of meeting their health needs – by using traditional practitioners, self-care, or the modern private sector. The health impacts are hard to determine. Among the policy consequences is a loss of authority by governments, as national health policy-making bodies. There is now a growing need to reassess roles, to develop realistic and coherent policies towards the private sector that will maximize its contribution to national health objectives while curbing its tendency to wasteful overpurchase of expensive technology. Central to this must be the concern to recreate an active role by government and to improve performance in the public sector. Unless these questions are addressed, government credibility as the architect of health policy will vanish.

In developing countries where there has been growth, trends in health sector reform and restructuring have been refined from single-thrust solutions such as user charges, community financing, or privatization and have increasingly become "package" approaches. Such packages often combine structural change (e.g., decentralization) with financing reform and, in varying degrees, attempt to improve efficiency in the government sector. Cost recovery for certain services for which people demonstrate willingness and ability to pay (e.g., drugs) will serve a useful function as long as the most vulnerable are not deterred from seeking care and the proceeds are ploughed back to improve and extend service availability. Some longer-term strategic deci-

sions, such as major capital decisions and human resources planning, risk neglect if "managed competition" overemphasizes the virtues of the market in these areas. Reform packages need to consider the distribution of health resources nationally, the scales of nongovernment and government subsectors, the most economical way of saving lives and reducing morbidity and disability, and the wider sharing of planning and regulatory responsibilities. The revitalization of the public sector in developing countries has tended to be a secondary concern in a period emphasizing nongovernment opportunities. In this respect there has emerged a major divergence of interest between developing and developed economies. Better performance in the public sector belongs high on the agenda for the developing countries in the coming years.

In developed countries, trends have been towards a convergence on a variety of managed market forms. There has been some success in the control (though not reduction) of total costs and in shifting regulatory procedures away from government. Attempts will continue to develop incentives for quality-based competition among providers of care, and to ensure that payment reflects workload. This will entail a movement away from salaried conditions of public service towards capitation-based payments, or to a mix of salary, capitation, and fee-for-service payments. Attempts are in progress to make first-level-care physicians budget holders not only for the primary but also for some of the referral needs of their patients.

Within insurance developments, trends have focused on the extension and better management of social insurance mechanisms rather than on large-scale reliance on the private health insurance market. A major concern is to prevent the exclusion of people at risk without producing unmanageable cost spirals.

In human resources for health, personal contact between client and health professional is and will always be central to health action. Therefore there will always be scope for innovation in the optimum deployment of the health workforce that goes beyond traditional divisions of professional responsibilities. One approach would be to look at the spectrum of skills required at a specific level of service and then identify who should be assigned.

Finally, in brief, the trends in research and development will generate new and improved preventive, diagnostic, therapeutic and enabling technologies, derived mainly from advances in the biological and physical sciences.

References

1. *Government Finance Statistics Yearbook*, vol. XIV. Washington, DC, International Monetary Fund, 1990.

2. McCarthy, F. & Fardoust, S. *Economic Issues for the 1990s*. Washington, DC, World Bank, 1991.

3. Ferroni, M. & Kanbur, R. *Poverty-conscious restructuring of public expenditure: social dimensions of adjustment in sub-Saharan Africa*. Washington, DC, World Bank, 1990 (Working Paper No. 9).

4. *Health care systems in transition: the search for efficiency*. Paris, Organisation for Economic Co-operation and Development, 1990.

5. Waddington, C. & Enyimayew, K. A price to pay, part 2. The impact of user charges in the Volta Region of Ghana. *International Journal of Health Planning and Management*, **5**: 287–312 (1990).

6. *Organization and financing of health care reforms in countries of central and eastern Europe*. Geneva, World Health Organization, 1991 (document WHO/DGO/91.1).

7. *Development cooperation in the 1990s*. Paris, Organization for Economic Co-operation and Development, 1989.

CHAPTER 5

Patterns and trends in health status

Mortality, morbidity, and disability

Mortality

It is generally recognized that good health is more than just the absence of disease and disability, although that is a vital component. Good health implies proper nutrition, adequate housing, and a social structure which allows the individual to lead a productive life and satisfy his or her basic physical, mental, and emotional needs. These components of positive health are, however, difficult to measure quantitatively. This chapter provides a summary of recent trends in health status as shown by mortality indicators and exploits available morbidity and disability data to better assess the situation with regard to specific diseases and conditions. The final section of the chapter provides an overview of some of the major determinants of ill health.

The data available on sickness, death, and disability is of variable quality, especially that from the developing countries. The best available estimates are used in the following assessment.

Years of research into the mortality of populations have led to the concept of an "epidemiological" or "mortality" transition, which is essentially a path to health development. Countries at the beginning of the transition have very high levels of death in children under 5, with infectious diseases as the leading cause. Subsequently, as these diseases are brought under control, under-5 mortality declines and the degenerative diseases emerge as leading causes of illness and death. At a final stage of the transition, as in the developed countries today, the traditional diseases of childhood are brought under control and the vast majority of deaths are postponed to very late in life.

Overall health status is well reflected by life expectancy at birth. Recent levels and trends in this indicator are shown in Fig. 5.1 for major development groups of countries. On average, a newborn baby in one of the developed countries

---

Global indicator 10
Life expectancy at birth, by sex, in all identifiable subgroups.

Fig. 5.1
Life expectancy at birth (both sexes) (global indicator 10), 1985 and 1991

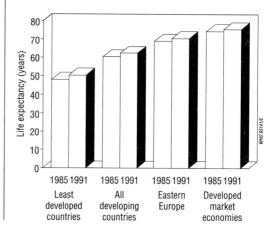

can expect to live 76 years, 26 years longer than a newborn in the least developed countries (see box). Life expectancy for other developing countries typically lies between these two values, being closer to the developed countries for the countries of east Asia and most of Latin America. Life expectancy in eastern Europe is, on average, just over 70 years.

The two situations described in the box represent the health extremes in the world of today. But there are countries within countries. Inhabitants of the highlands of tropical countries do not get nearly as much malaria as those in the swampy lowlands. Adults who live in the urban areas of Japan are significantly less likely to suffer from stroke than those in rural areas.

Parts of certain cities in some developed countries have vaccination coverage rates lower than those of some developing countries. Be they in developed or developing countries, the unfortunate inhabitants of the slums in many cities have a life expectancy shorter than the national average.

And there are peoples within peoples. Among the 250 million inhabitants of the United States are thousands of Americans whose life expectancy and other health parameters are much lower than those of the rest of the population. Conversely, in even the least developed countries there are some people who are better educated and financially better off, whose prospects for a long and healthy life approach those of people in the richest countries.

Worldwide, life expectancy has increased by between one and two years over the past 5 years,[1] with the global average currently 65 years. Females outlive males by seven years in the developed countries, and by two years in the least developed countries. This widening gap in survival between the sexes as mortality decreases is primarily due to men having been the first to expose themselves to risk factors for chronic diseases, particularly cigarette smoking.

As expected, virtually all developed countries, as well as those in eastern Europe, attained an average level of life expectancy in excess of 70 years (the single exception being South Africa). On the other hand, no least developed

---

1. This information is based on UN Population Division estimates for the 5-year (mid-year) periods 1980–1985, 1985–1990, and 1990–1995.

The fortunate one in eight

A baby girl born in one of the richest countries in 1990 can expect to live to the age of 81, five years longer than a baby boy born in that country the same year. As she grows up she is assured of adequate nutrition, hygienic living conditions, adequate schooling, and advanced medical care. She will receive full vaccination against all childhood diseases at the appropriate age and the proper intervals. She will probably not marry until she reaches her twenties and will then have one or two children, properly spaced, delivered in hospital after regular prenatal checkups. The greatest dangers to her health in her middle years will be the risk of an accident at home or while she is out driving, or a particularly virulent influenza epidemic. As she enters old age she will be liable to develop cardiovascular disease or cancer, but will survive the first attacks of these with little disability because of excellent medical care and rehabilitation services. She will receive good institutional care in her old age. She will spend on average, including government assistance, the equivalent of US$ 1000 on her health every year.

Seventeen million babies, one-eighth of the world total, were born in the developed nations in 1990, and most of them will grow up to enjoy conditions of life and health similar to those of this fortunate little girl.

The most deprived one in seven

A baby girl born on the same day in the most disadvantaged of the least developed countries can expect to live barely 43 years, three years more than a baby boy born the same year. Her problems begin before birth, since her mother is likely to be in poor health. If she is born in south Asia, the baby has a one-in-four chance of being underweight, a greater chance of dying in infancy than a baby boy, and a high probability of being malnourished throughout childhood. She has a one-in-five chance of dying before her first birthday and a one-in-three chance of dying before her fifth. In some African countries her chance of being vaccinated is less than one in five. She will be brought up in inadequate housing under insanitary conditions contributing to diarrhoeal disease, cholera, and tuberculosis. She will have a less than one in four chance of ever getting enough schooling to learn how to read and write. She may be circumcised at puberty, with consequent effects on her life as a woman and a mother. She will marry in her teens and may have 10 or more children, close together, unless she dies in childbirth before that. Ancient traditions will prevent her from eating certain nutritious foods during her pregnancies, when she most needs building up, and dangerous practices such as using an unsterile knife to cut the umbilical cord and placing cow dung on the stump may kill some of her babies with tetanus. In fact, 3 or 4 of her children will die before the age of five because she has no access to prenatal care, or antitetanus vaccination, or a trained midwife, or medical care for the child. Neither will she have access to family planning facilities or the means to protect herself against AIDS.

She will be in constant danger of infectious disease from contaminated water at the place where she bathes, washes clothes, and collects drinking-water, and from parasites carried by insects. She will be chronically anaemic from poor nutrition, malaria, and intestinal parasites. As well as caring for her family she will work hard in the fields, suffering from repeated attacks of fever, fatigue, and infected cuts from thorns or farm implements. If she survives into old age she will suffer the same afflictions as women in the rich countries: cardiovascular disease and cancer. To these she will succumb quickly, because she has no access to proper medical care and rehabilitation. Her country has less than US$ 1 a year to spend on her health; she cannot afford to pay anything herself.

Twenty million babies, one-seventh of the world total, were born in the least developed countries in 1990, and too many of them will grow up in miserable conditions of life and health. For every newborn in the affluent countries, there is one in the least developed countries. Equity demands that the situation of these deprived infants be improved without delay.

---

country has yet achieved this level, and only two have a life expectancy at birth in the range 60–69 years. The majority of least developed countries still exhibit a life expectancy below 50 years. Among the remaining group of developing countries, about half have achieved a life expectancy of 60–69 years, with another 18 countries already enjoying a life expectancy of 70 years or more, comparable to the developed countries. Twenty developing countries (excluding the least developed) still have yet to at-

tain an average life expectancy of 60 years or more. This distribution of countries is roughly the same for both males and females.

Perinatal, infant, and child mortality

Of the 140 million babies born each year, almost 4 million die within hours or days from perinatal causes. These include neonatal tetanus (560 000 deaths in 1990), birth asphyxia, birth trauma, prematurity, congenital anomalies, neonatal pneumonia, sepsis, and meningitis. Contributing to these causes are malnutrition, other infections, and the consequences of unregulated fertility and closely spaced pregnancies. Other major causes of death below the age of one year are acute respiratory infections and pneumonia, diarrhoea, measles, pertussis, and malaria. Approximately 95% of these deaths occur in the developing countries.

In countries where the prevalence of infectious and parasitic disease is still high, about one-half of all deaths typically occur before the age of five. Two-thirds of these occur among infants, and the remaining third at ages 1–4 years from the same six diseases mentioned above as being common causes of infant death.[1]

Every year over 1500 million episodes of diarrhoea and more than 40 million episodes of pneumonia occur in this age group. Millions of deaths result and millions of dollars or their equivalent in health care are spent; children who survive suffer from malnutrition or their existing malnutrition gets worse.

Not surprisingly, the relative differences in health status identified from the data on life expectancy mirror those from infant and child mortality. Thus the infant mortality rate for the least developed countries in 1988–90 is almost 120 per 1000, or 8–9 times higher than the rate for developed countries (Fig. 5.2). Globally, the infant mortality rate has fallen from 76 per 1000 in 1983–1985 to 68 per 1000 in 1988–1990.

Improved education for girls and women, together with enhanced access to health care, has a positive effect on maternal and infant mortality. In two villages in Nigeria, for example, life expectancy at birth for infants of illiterate mothers was increased by 20% when the sole

---

Global indicator 9
The infant mortality rate (IMR), maternal mortality rate (MMR), and probability of dying before the age of 5 years (q5), in all identifiable subgroups.

Fig. 5.2
Infant mortality rate (global indicator 9.1), 1985 and 1991

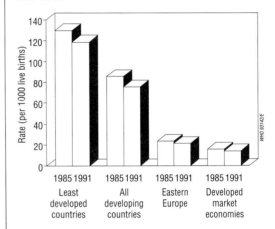

---

intervention was access by their mothers to health facilities; by 33% when illiterate mothers participated in relevant educational activities; and by 87% through the synergistic effect of both interventions. Perinatal mortality, which accounts for approximately half of all infant mortality, is also sharply reduced by maternal education.

A similar pattern of deaths is seen in children below age 5 (Fig. 5.3). In the least developed countries almost 200 children out of every 1000 born alive will die before reaching age 5, compared with less than 20 in the developed countries. The under-5 mortality rate for the remaining group of developing countries is about 120 per 1000 live births.

In all developed countries except South Africa, the infant mortality rate is below 20 for 1000 live births, as it is in five of the eight countries of eastern Europe. On the contrary, infant mortality rates of 100 per 1000 or higher are still

---

1. Estimates of combined infant and child mortality, such as the under-5 mortality rate, are generally more reliable than separate estimates of infant and child mortality. Therefore, to monitor levels of premature mortality in countries, two indicators are used, namely the infant mortality rate and the under-5 mortality rate (i.e., the probability of dying before age 5). Both of these indicators are expressed per 1000 live births.

observed in the majority of least developed countries, with only seven of them having a rate below this level, and only one (Cape Verde) with a rate below 50 per 1000 live births. Infant mortality rates for the remainder of the developing countries are virtually evenly distributed into two groups: 50 per 1000 and above, or less than 50 per 1000. Indeed, 11 developing countries have already attained an IMR below 20 per 1000 live births, the level of the developed world.

The distribution of countries within development groups is roughly the same when the under-5 mortality rate is used to measure child mortality. In virtually all the least developed countries for which estimates are available, at least 15% of children die before their fifth birthday. For the remainder of the developing countries, the probability of child death is much lower, with 29 countries having an under-5 mortality rate less than 5% and another 22 having a probability of child death between 5% and 10%.

Comparing child mortality during the last 15 years, one finds that significant reductions in child deaths have been recorded during the more recent period in several areas of the developing world. In northern Africa, the rate of decline since 1975 is twice that of the earlier period and in Latin America it is 50% greater. In contrast, for sub-Saharan Africa the pace of decline in the recent period has slowed and is only about half as great as in the earlier period. Where significant improvements in child survival have been recorded, they probably reflect the gains in women's educational attainment, improvements in access to and delivery of health services including oral rehydration and vaccination, and the success of family planning programmes, which have reduced the number of births and lengthened the interval between them (1).

Although the adolescent ages correspond to that period of life when the risk of death is at its lowest, death rates are still unacceptably high in some regions of the world. The principal causes of death in adolescence are accidents, acute respiratory disease, and malaria in developing

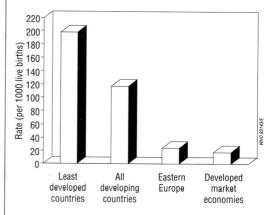

Fig. 5.3

Under-5 mortality rate (probability of dying before age 5) (global indicator 9.3), 1991

countries. In developed countries, accidents and violence account for over half of all adolescent mortality, with childhood cancers a significant cause as well. Moreover, in a number of developed countries, suicide rates among adolescents have increased markedly in recent years, reflecting the myriad social pressures on young people and their increased expectations (2).

Maternal mortality

Over 500 000 women die each year from causes related to pregnancy and childbirth. Maternal mortality in 1988 varied from about 737 per 100 000 live births in the least developed countries to about 34 per 100 000 live births in the developed market economies (Fig. 5.4). Although most maternal deaths take place in southern Asia (this being the region where most births occur), pregnancies and childbirth have become somewhat safer for women in most of Asia and parts of Latin America. The risks a woman undergoes when she becomes pregnant and/or gives birth are highest in eastern, middle and western Africa. A woman in sub-Saharan Africa who becomes pregnant is 75 times more likely to die as a result than a woman in western Europe. In countries where the risk is highest, such as Somalia or the Gambia, the difference is 100-fold.

The direct causes of these deaths vary little from country to country. The five major ones are haemorrhage, infection, unsafe abortion, hypertension, and obstructed labour. Many women who survive these complications are left with serious, chronic disabilities such as vesicovaginal fistula, uterine prolapse, and secondary infertility. The knowledge and technology needed to prevent the majority of these deaths have existed for years; they are neither sophisticated nor expensive, they merely need to be applied.

Little is known about the trends in maternal mortality in developing countries. Indeed, it is only since the mid-1980s that the dimensions of the problem have been recognized. Maternal mortality was not included as a global indicator in the previous global health evaluation. In a number of countries or population groups, where death registration and death certification are haphazard, deficient, or absent, when specific studies are done, maternal mortality is frequently found to be high.

A number of countries have succeeded in reducing maternal mortality rates through a combined strategy of improving the status of women, increasing coverage with family planning services, increasing the number of well-trained personnel to care for women during pregnancy and birth, and setting up networks of supporting hospitals for referral. Using such a strategy, for example, Sri Lanka has succeeded, over a 25-year period, in reducing maternal mortality from 500 to only 80 per 100 000 live births.

Mortality in the elderly

As the mortality transition progresses, more and more people are surviving to older ages. In Sweden, for example, about 80% of girls born in the early 1950s could expect to live to age 65. Today this proportion has risen to 90%. Similar gains have been achieved in other developed countries as well. As a result life expectancy at age 65 has increased significantly in many countries.

Fig. 5.4
Maternal mortality rate (global indicator 9.2), 1991

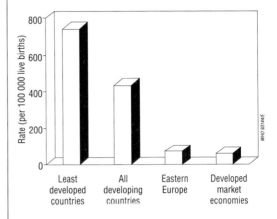

For the developed countries, male life expectancy at age 65 has increased on average by 1.6 years, i.e., from 13.0 in 1960 to 14.6 years in the late 1980s. For females, the gains in life expectancy at age 65 have been even more impressive, rising by 3.3 years from an average of 15.2 to 18.5 years over the same period.

Although life expectancy of the elderly has generally increased, it is not at all clear whether sickness and disability among them have declined in parallel with mortality rates. Available evidence suggests that the extra years of life that have been gained in the past two decades have largely been years tarnished by disability, which reduces the quality of life and increases the demand for health and social services. The major causes of disability and handicap among the elderly include arthritis, deafness, blindness, and Alzheimer's disease and related neurological disorders. To these may be added the mental problems caused by social isolation and depression.

Sex differentials in mortality

The number of boys born is slightly greater than the number of girls. Yet in most societies, the number of women surviving into old age is much greater than the number of men.

Studies of the trends and patterns of these sex differences in life expectancy from several European countries and a few least developed countries are consistent with the following sequence of events, although they do not prove that this is what is actually happening. The factors affecting life span fall into two broad groups, one being genetic and biological and the other social, environmental, economic, and cultural. The genetic and biological factors seem to be unequal between the sexes. In the least developed countries, with their high mortality and low longevity, sociocultural and environmental factors often cancel out the biological advantage of being female, so that the life expectancy at birth of males may in some cases exceed that of females. But as a country develops and its environment improves, with better hygiene, nutrition, health care, education, and living standards, the disadvantage to women is overcome

and their biological advantage is asserted. In a third stage, the detrimental effects of an affluent society start to take over, with unbalanced nutrition, industrial health hazards, traffic accidents, and alcohol and tobacco abuse. These at first affect males, because social taboos discourage these behaviours among women, and the gender gap widens, but as women progressively take up accident-prone jobs outside the home and the noxious habits first adopted by men, the gap can be expected to narrow again (*3*).

Specific diseases and conditions

Each year, about 50 million people die throughout the world. Over the past six years, the fall in the death rate has been cancelled out by the rise in the population. Of these 50 million, about 6.8 million deaths are registered in the developed market economies, 4.2 million in eastern Eu-

Fig. 5.5

Estimated annual number of deaths by cause in developing and developed countries, 1990

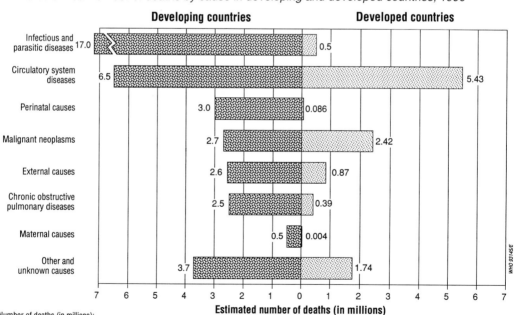

Number of deaths (in millions):
Total: 49.9
Developing countries: 38.5
Developed countries: 11.4

rope, 7 million in the group of least developed countries and 32 million elsewhere in the developing world. Reliable data on causes of death are available to WHO for only about one-third of these, mainly from the developed countries. None the less, on the basis of community studies and health services information, the approximate distribution of deaths by cause for the developing countries can be derived (Fig. 5.5) (4). In view of the significance of under-5 mortality in the developing world, estimates for this population group are presented separately in Table 5.1.

Between 1985 and 1990, the number of infant and child deaths in the developing countries fell from 13.5 million to 12.9 million. This decline was primarily due to the marked reduction in deaths from measles (2 million to 880 000), pertussis (600 000 to 360 000) and neonatal tetanus (800 000 to 560 000), reflecting the success of the Expanded Programme on Immunization in the 1980s. Unfortunately, deaths from

Table 5.1

Estimated causes of death among children under 5 years of age in developing countries, 1985 and 1990

Cause of death category	1990		1985	
	Number of deaths (in thousands)	%	Number of deaths (in thousands)	%
1. Acute respiratory infections (ARI) alone (mostly pneumonia)*	3 560	27.6	3 300	24.4
2. Diarrhoea alone	3 000	23.3	3 000	22.2
3. Birth asphyxia	860	6.7	760	5.6
4. Malaria	800	6.2	750	5.6
5. Neonatal tetanus	560	4.3	800	5.9
6. ARI – measles	480	3.7	1 100	8.1
7. Congenital anomalies	450	3.5	400	3.0
8. Birth trauma	430	3.3	380	2.8
9. Prematurity	430	3.3	380	2.8
10. Neonatal sepsis and meningitis	300	2.3	180	1.3
11. Tuberculosis	300	2.3	300	2.2
12. ARI – pertussis	260	2.0	400	3.0
13. Measles alone	220	1.7	500	3.7
14. Accidents	200	1.6	200	1.5
15. Diarrhoea – measles	180	1.4	400	3.0
16. Pertussis alone	100	0.8	200	1.5
17. All other causes	770	6.0	450	3.3
Total	12 900	100.0	13 500	100.0
ARI total (1,6,12)	4 300	33.3	4 800	35.6
Neonatal and perinatal, total (3,5,7,8,9,10*)	3 830	29.7	3 700	27.4
Diarrhoea total (2,15)	3 180	24.7	3 400	25.2
Vaccine-preventable, total (5,6,11,12,13,15,16)	2 100	16.3	3 700	27.4
Measles total (6,13,15)	880	6.8	2 000	14.8
Pertussis total (12,16)	360	2.8	600	4.4

* Including 800 000 deaths from neonatal pneumonia.

neonatal and perinatal causes and acute respiratory infections (mostly pneumonia) increased, which is why the total reduction in deaths is less than the reduction due to immunization. The annual number of diarrhoea-related deaths fell by about 200 000 and currently accounts for about one-quarter of all child deaths. Another quarter is attributable to acute respiratory infections, primarily pneumonia, including 800 000 neonatal deaths. Malaria is thought to cause another 800 000 child deaths each year. A further 3 million deaths result from conditions common to the perinatal period (excluding the 800 000 neonatal deaths from pneumonia mentioned above).

Among adults worldwide, deaths are mainly due to the chronic diseases, which have also emerged as leading causes of death in a number of developing countries. Cardiovascular diseases claim about 6 million lives every year in the developing world, as many as in the developed countries and eastern Europe combined. Similarly, cancer now claims more victims in developing countries (2.7 million deaths per year) than in the developed world (2.4 million). A similar number die each year in the developing world from the chronic obstructive lung diseases, primarily chronic bronchitis and emphysema (4).

At the same time, the infectious and parasitic diseases continue to pose serious risks to adult health in developing countries. Tuberculosis claims around 3 million lives each year, 90% of which are among the adult population. Pneumonia is the cause of about 2 million adult deaths each year in developing countries, and another million or so die from diarrhoeal diseases. Maternal mortality remains a significant health problem in many parts of the developing world, with 500 000 women dying each year from complications of pregnancy and the puerperium. Other major health risks for adults include malaria, schistosomiasis, hepatitis B, and AIDS, each of which accounts for several hundred thousand adult deaths each year.

Thus the constellation of health problems that affect people throughout the world includes infectious and parasitic diseases, noncommunicable diseases, mental and neurological problems, injuries, and disability. These affect populations in varying proportions depending on where they are in the epidemiological transition; typically, developing countries have a larger proportion of communicable diseases and developed countries a larger proportion of noncommunicable diseases.

Infectious and parasitic diseases

Taken together, this category of diseases accounts for about 17 million deaths, or almost half of all deaths occurring in developing countries (4). However, the associated illness affects substantially more people and perhaps better reflects the public health dimension of these diseases. A brief overview is given below, with the diseases ranked approximately in order of the amount of illness they cause.

Intestinal parasitic infections. The current prevalence of these parasites is: 1000 million infections with roundworms (*Ascaris*), 900 million with hookworm (*Ancylostoma*) and 500 million with whipworm (*Trichuris*); they are thus among the most common infections in the world. The protozoan parasite *Giardia lamblia* is distributed worldwide, affecting almost one in every three people. Although most adults show no symptoms, giardiasis is an important cause of growth retardation and the main parasitic cause of acute diarrhoea in small children. *Entamoeba histolytica*, the protozoan parasite that causes amoebiasis, causes much diarrhoea and is the second most important cause of death due to protozoan infections globally, after malaria. Strongyloidiasis, caused by a worm, is associated with severe malnutrition and malabsorption. Chronic infections with mixtures of these parasites affect the growth and even the academic progress of children throughout the developing world.

Diarrhoeal diseases. These remain a major cause of morbidity and mortality in infants and young children in developing countries. A child under five years of age in the developing world suffers from, on average, 2.8 episodes of diarrhoea per year. This results in 1500 million episodes of illness, and more than 3 million deaths each year in children aged under five. In addition to acute watery diarrhoea which accounts for the largest proportion of these deaths, dysentery and persistent diarrhoea are also important problems. An additional one million deaths a year occur in adults. Diarrhoea cases in many parts of the world still account for one-third or more of hospital admissions, and they often receive expensive intravenous fluids, unnecessary antibiotics, and "anti-diarrhoeal" drugs, instead of effective and inexpensive oral rehydration salts or fluids available in the home, thereby creating an unnecessarily heavy burden on limited national health budgets.

In addition, outbreaks of cholera, more commonly affecting older children and adults, have severe socioeconomic consequences beyond the health sector. The seventh recorded cholera pandemic, after 30 years of westward spread from its origins in the Far East, reached the Americas at the beginning of 1991, where it produced a spectacular epidemic in Peru which affected almost a quarter of a million people in the first six months, and spread to neighbouring countries (Fig. 5.6). Cholera may well become endemic in the long term, thus posing a threat to the whole of Latin America and the Caribbean.

Acute respiratory infections. On average, everyone in the world gets two attacks per year of the common cold. In some cases, this develops into something more serious. The total number of episodes of acute respiratory infections in young children throughout the world is 2000 million a year. The high incidence is also reflected in the statistics of treatment facilities, in which acute respiratory infections account for more than one-third of paediatric visits and hospitalizations in most countries.

Acute respiratory infections are now estimated to be the first cause of childhood mortality in developing countries. They are responsible for 4.3 million deaths annually. Almost 20% or 800 000 of these deaths are due to pneumonia in the neonatal period. About 10% of the other deaths are caused by complications after measles or pertussis infections, and could be prevented by immunization. Malnutrition and low birthweight are important contributory factors to the mortality toll; the gradual reduction in the prevalence of these risk factors will contribute to the prevention of deaths from pneumonia. However, case management is the central strategy for making immediate impact on the mortality from acute respiratory infections that cannot be prevented by immunization.

There are no global figures on influenza morbidity but a moderately severe influenza season can affect one-tenth of the population. Apart from being a real death threat to the elderly and people with lowered resistance, influenza epidemics are associated with enormous social costs in terms of disrupted public services, interrupted education and increased medical care.

Vaccine-preventable diseases. The incidence of the target diseases of the Expanded Programme on Immunization in 1989 was: measles 49 million cases, pertussis 45.8 million, tetanus (all ages) 1.5 million, poliomyelitis 190 000. The urgent need to raise immunization coverage levels further is underlined by the continuing occurrence each year of some 1.6 million preventable deaths from measles, neonatal tetanus and whooping cough, some 120 000 cases of paralytic poliomyelitis and 1–2 million deaths attributable to hepatitis B infection.

Since some of these infections cause death through diarrhoeal or respiratory symptoms, the figures given here are included in those shown in the sections above.

Almost all countries have adopted the new disease-reduction targets for the decade of the 1990s: the reduction of measles deaths by 95%,

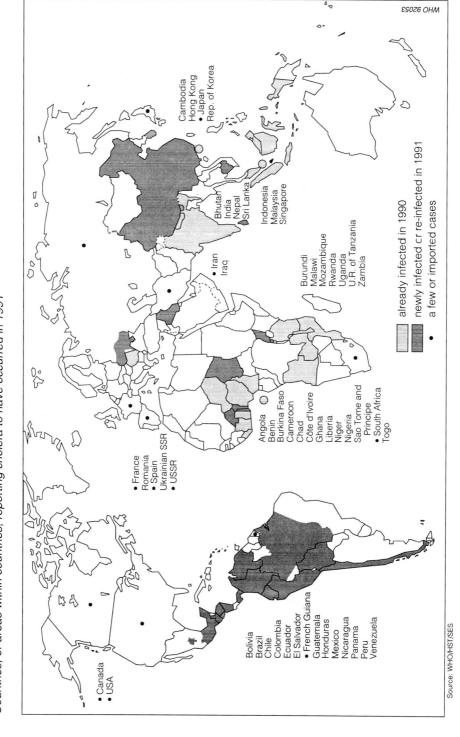

Fig. 5.6
Countries, or areas within countries, reporting cholera to have occurred in 1991

the elimination of neonatal tetanus by 1995, the eradication of poliomyelitis by the year 2000, and the achievement and maintenance of a 90% immunization rate for the six diseases for infants and the same rate for immunization against tetanus for women of child-bearing age.

Skin infections. One of the commonest reasons why people go to the health services for treatment is for skin infections due to bacterial, fungal, or arthropod (scabies) attack. These are a special problem in tropical areas and among people living under poor hygienic conditions.

Sexually transmitted diseases. These continue to be among the most frequent infectious conditions worldwide, with a constantly high incidence. The annual incidence of the major sexually transmitted diseases is 250 million, as follows: trichomoniasis, 120 million cases; genital chlamydial infections, 50 million; genital human papillomavirus infection, 30 million; gonorrhoea, 25 million; genital herpes, 20 million; infectious syphilis, 3.5 million; chancroid, 2 million. In addition, over 1 million people a year are newly infected with HIV, the virus causing AIDS, and this number is increasing.

In the developed world the rates of many bacterial sexually transmitted diseases have stabilized, but the incidence appears to be increasing in the developing world. Chlamydial and in particular viral infections, among them HIV infection and its consequence AIDS, are increasingly prevalent in all areas of the world. Reasons for the high incidence of sexually transmitted diseases, especially in the developing world, should be sought in a number of variables, in particular urbanization, unemployment, economic hardship, and a loosening of traditional restraints on sexual activity, as well as the emergence of antibiotic-resistant strains of microorganisms. In addition, the population pyramid is heavily weighted with individuals in the most sexually active age-groups.

While infection rates are similar in men and women, it is women and children who bear the major brunt of the complications and serious sequelae of sexually transmitted diseases. A large proportion of infertility and ectopic pregnancy is a consequence of pelvic inflammatory disease and is thus preventable. Sexually transmitted diseases in pregnant women can result in prematurity, stillbirth, and neonatal infection. In many areas 1–5% of newborns are at risk of gonococcal ophthalmia neonatorum (a blinding disease); congenital syphilis causes up to a quarter of perinatal mortality in a few countries.

Schistosomiasis. Since 1985, two additional countries have notified WHO that schistosomiasis is now endemic, increasing the total to 76 countries. Schistosomiasis is endemic in 27 of the least developed countries. There are 600 million people exposed, among whom 200 million are infected and 20 million have serious symptoms. Since the peak prevalence and intensity of infection is among the young (10–19 year olds), they bear the main burden. The sequelae of heavy infection, in the form of liver and urinary tract disease, including bladder cancer, which is the leading cause of cancer death in Egyptian males 20–44 years of age, affect the most economically productive sector of the population.

As rural migration to the towns continues unabated, the urban transmission of schistosomiasis is no longer an exception in large cities from Nouakchott (Mauritania) to Luanda (Angola) on the west coast of Africa, and in the north-east of Brazil. Schistosomiasis is increasingly reported in refugees in Ethiopia and Somalia (transmission of *Schistosoma mansoni* has now been confirmed in Somalia), Cameroon, Chad, Malawi, Mozambique, and Zimbabwe.

Drancunculiasis (guinea-worm disease) has been a major health risk for millions of people in Africa and the Indian subcontinent. Effective national eradication programmes and the International Drinking Water Supply and Sanitation Decade (1981–1990) have succeeded in reducing the estimated annual global number of cases from 10 million in 1985 to less than 3 million in 1991. While 100 million people remain at risk of infection, the life cycle of the parasite offers a unique possibility of eliminating the disease with simple technology. The human host acquires the parasite by drinking contaminated water, and eradication depends largely on the provision of safe water: village pumps in endemic areas, filtering of surface water where piped water is unavailable and destruction of the cyclops, the intermediate host of the worm. The goal of global eradication by 1995 set by WHO Member States at the World Health Assembly in May 1991 is feasible if national commitment and dedication to the programme is maintained.

Malaria. The malaria situation worldwide is not improving and in many places is deteriorating compared with 10 years ago. More than 2000 million people, almost half the world's population, are exposed to varying degrees of malaria risk in some 100 countries and areas. In countries of Africa south of the Sahara about 100 million clinical cases of malaria occur every year, with close to 1 million deaths. During the period under review, epidemics or serious outbreaks occurred in several normally low-incidence highland areas of Africa, particularly in Botswana, Burundi, Ethiopia, Madagascar, Rwanda, Swaziland, and Zambia. In other parts of the world, while malaria remains under control in most developed and stable areas, the situation is dramatically deteriorating in all frontier areas of economic development, such as those with intensified exploitation of natural resources (agriculture, mining, etc.), in jungle areas or areas burdened with problems of civil war and other conflicts, illegal trade, and mass movements of refugees. Outside Africa, most of the 5.2 million cases reported to WHO in 1989 originated in only 25 of the countries with endemic malaria. Half of all cases were recorded in India and Brazil; a further quarter were from Thailand, Sri Lanka, Afghanistan, Viet Nam, China, and Myanmar (in decreasing order).

Tuberculosis. Tuberculosis is one of the most widespread infections. Approximately

1700 million people, or one-third of the world's population, are at risk of developing the disease. Whereas in otherwise healthy people this risk is fairly low, it is markedly increased in certain conditions such as malnutrition and especially HIV infection. In 1990, there were 8 million new cases, of which 7.6 million were in developing countries. Tuberculosis caused about 3 million deaths and therefore was the leading cause of death attributable to a single infectious pathogen. In the developing countries four-fifths of both incidence and mortality were in the economically most productive age-groups (15–59 years), in which tuberculosis accounted for over one-quarter of all avoidable deaths.

Since 1985 the incidence of tuberculosis has started to increase in some developed countries and in many sub-Saharan and Caribbean countries as a result of the association of tuberculosis and HIV infection. HIV infection is by far the highest risk factor for tuberculosis infection to progress to disease: of those infected with both tuberculosis and HIV, at least one-third, and probably an even higher proportion, will develop tuberculous disease. By the end of 1990, already more than 3 million people were dually infected, of whom 2.4 million were in sub-Saharan African countries.

In the developing countries most affected by HIV infection, the tuberculosis problem is assuming dramatic dimensions: in certain areas the numbers of diagnosed cases have doubled over the past five years, causing increased demands for diagnostic services, drugs, and hospital beds, which can barely be met by the existing health care systems. Since the HIV epidemic is still in its ascending phase and tuberculosis normally does not develop until several years after HIV infection, and since the increase in incidence will entail an increase in transmission of tuberculosis, the situation will worsen tremendously unless drastic control measures are taken forthwith. Asian countries should be on the alert; in many of these countries tuberculosis infection is even more common than in

Africa, and HIV infection is making dramatic inroads.

Mosquito-borne viral diseases. Dengue and dengue haemorrhagic fever continue to spread and now occur in most of the tropical world – in 1988 they were reported in five continents. Between 30 and 60 million infections occur annually, and the condition is a leading cause of death in under-fives in some east Asian countries.

Japanese encephalitis is endemic in Asia from India all the way to Japan. About 40 000 cases occur each year. It is associated with a high case-fatality rate: 10–40% die and among survivors 10–30% have severe neurological sequelae. A highly effective but expensive vaccine has been added to the routine childhood immunization programme in some affected areas.

Yellow fever has been extraordinarily active during the period beginning in 1986, with thousands of cases and deaths reported, mostly in Africa (mainly Nigeria). The Americas also experienced an exceptionally high number of case reports in this period: 629 cases and 540 deaths. Surveys have shown that reported cases represent only a fraction of the true numbers. A cheap and highly effective vaccine has been added to the routine childhood immunization programme in several endemic African countries.

Trypanosomiasis. Ninety-five million individuals, one-fifth of the Latin American population, are at risk of contracting infection by the parasite *Trypanosoma cruzi*. Sixteen to 18 million people are actually infected and can develop either of the main chronic clinical forms in the next 10 years: the cardiac form, 5 million cases, and the digestive form 1.5 million cases. Between 2% (Sao Paulo, Brazil) and 63% (Santa Cruz, Bolivia) of blood donations in blood banks of cities in the endemic countries are positive for *T. cruzi* infection.

Fifty million people live in the tsetse fly belt of tropical Africa and are at risk of African trypanosomiasis, but only 10% of these are under regular surveillance or have access to diagnostic facilities, so the 25 000 cases reported annually are a serious underestimate. The mortality rate is 100% if not treated.

Leishmaniasis. This parasitic disease spread by minute biting flies is far more abundant and of greater public health importance than was previously recognized. It is found in 80 countries in four continents, its overall prevalence is 12 million cases, and 390 million people are at risk. Worldwide there is an increasing number of cases and a more widespread geographical distribution, the disease being reported from previously non-endemic areas. Economic and demographic circumstances that contribute to increased prevalence include: new agro-industrial projects, large-scale migration of populations, unplanned urbanization, and man-made environmental changes.

Hepatitis. More than 2000 million persons, or 2 out of every 5 people on earth, are infected with the hepatitis B virus. About 300 million of them are chronically infected carriers, one-quarter of whom are at high risk of serious illness and eventual death from cirrhosis of the liver and primary liver cancer. It is estimated that more than one million deaths per year occur from the sequelae of these infections. Virtually all are preventable, since safe and effective vaccines have been available since 1982, and have been used in more than 70 million individuals. More than 72 countries have included the vaccine in their regular health services or are planning to do so in the near future. In 22 countries, primarily in the western Pacific and eastern Mediterranean, the vaccine is either routinely offered to all infants as part of the services of the Expanded Programme on Immunization or will be included in this programme in the very near future.

Rabies. Canine rabies continues to exist in 87 countries or territories of the world and accounts for 99% of all human rabies cases. The human death toll in developing countries is 30 000 cases in Asia, 5000 in Africa and 300 in

Latin America. Globally each year 5.6 million people require rabies treatment because of animal bites.

Leprosy. In 1990 the total number of registered cases in the world was 3.7 million, giving a global prevalence rate of 7.1 patients per 10 000 population. The total number of newly detected cases was 576 361, with a global detection rate of 1.1 cases per 10 000 population. South-east Asia has the greatest leprosy problem, with almost three-quarters of the total cases in the world; the regional prevalence and detection rates of 20.5 and 3.7 patients per 10 000 population, respectively, are also the highest when compared with other regions. The magnitude of the problem in Africa and the Americas is much less, while Europe, the Middle East, China and east Asia together have less than 10% of the total registered cases.

The WHO strategy for leprosy control is based on the implementation of multidrug therapy regimens. This strategy has been adopted by all endemic countries during the past five years, and the resulting progress in the control of leprosy has been remarkable. For the first time, there has been a reduction in the number of registered cases from 5.4 million in 1985 to 3.7 million in 1990, representing a decrease of 31.5%.

Endemic treponematoses. Globally, there are more than 2.5 million cases of yaws, endemic syphilis and pinta, three-quarters of them children; more than 100 million children are at risk of these disabling and disfiguring infections. The situation is particularly alarming in west and central Africa where 1.2 million children are infected with endemic treponemal diseases. Drastic increases of nonvenereal endemic syphilis are reported from the Sahel countries, with 15–40% of children showing serological evidence of past or present infection and 2–20% suffering from infectious lesions. Reports of disease outbreaks continue to come from the Thai/Malaysian border area.

HIV infection and AIDS. HIV infection and AIDS are pandemic worldwide. However,

they have not affected the world's population uniformly (Fig. 5.7). Extensive spread appears, in retrospect, to have commenced in the late 1970s or early 1980s primarily in populations of: (1) homosexual or bisexual men and injecting drug users in certain urban areas of the Americas, Australasia, and western Europe; and (2) men and women with multiple sexual partners in parts of the Caribbean and eastern and central Africa.

Two HIV viruses are recognized, HIV-1 and HIV-2. Worldwide, the predominant virus is HIV-1. Extensive spread of HIV-2 occurred through the 1980s, principally in west Africa. The modes of transmission of HIV-1 and HIV-2 are similar, and AIDS cases resulting from HIV-1 or HIV-2 infections appear to be clinically indistinguishable. In this chapter, the abbreviation HIV is used to refer to HIV-1.

Studies to date indicate that about 50% of adults infected with HIV will develop AIDS within 10 years of infection. Few data are available beyond 10 years, but it is expected that the vast majority of HIV-infected persons will develop AIDS eventually. No major differences have so far been found in the rate of progression from HIV to AIDS by geographical area, sex, or race. In infants born infected with HIV, the progression to AIDS is more rapid than in adults.

Virtually all persons diagnosed as having AIDS die within a few years. Survival after diagnosis has been increasing in developed countries from an average of less than 1 year to about 1–2 years. However, survival time for AIDS cases in developing countries remains short – an estimated 6 months or less. Longer survival appears to be directly related to the routine use of antiviral drugs, the use of prophylactic drugs for some opportunistic infections (e.g., pneumonia due to *Pneumocystis*), and to a better overall quality of health care.

By late 1991, more than 400 000 AIDS cases had been reported to WHO, but when underdiagnosis, underreporting, and delays in reporting are taken into account, more than one million AIDS cases may have occurred in adults worldwide to date. In addition, by mid-1991 more than 500 000 paediatric AIDS cases resulting from perinatal transmission may have occurred, with more than 90% of this total in sub-Saharan Africa. Thus, the cumulative global total of AIDS cases by early 1991 stands at more than 1.5 million.

As of mid-1991, at least 8–10 million HIV infections have occurred in adults since the beginning of the pandemic, and about one million children have been born infected with HIV. For the year 2000, WHO projects cumulative totals of 40 million HIV infections, including over 10 million children, and close to 10 million adult AIDS cases.

AIDS has become increasingly a problem of the developing countries, which accounted for half the global total of HIV infections in 1985 and two-thirds in 1990, with the infection transmitted increasingly through heterosexual intercourse (50% of HIV infections in 1985, 60% in 1990, 75–80% by the year 2000) (5).

Noncommunicable diseases

Noncommunicable diseases, e.g., cardiovascular and chronic respiratory diseases, diabetes, and cancer, are a real epidemic today in the developed countries, being responsible for three-quarters of all deaths, and are an emerging epidemic in the developing world. While some developing countries remain burdened primarily with the problems of hunger and malnutrition and communicable diseases, in other countries in that group there have been increases in the occurrence of chronic diseases.

Mortality data from Chile and Finland illustrate this trend. In Finland, the proportion of deaths from noncommunicable diseases was 70% in 1954 and rose slowly to 79.5% in 1986, reflecting its economic development and age structure. As predicted by the demographic changes associated with its development, Chile displayed a more pronounced trend: only 40%

of deaths from noncommunicable diseases in 1954, with a rapid increase to 68% in 1988. Sixteen countries in east and south-east Asia are already reporting more deaths from noncommunicable diseases than from communicable diseases, and there are similar trends in other developing regions.

The major noncommunicable diseases are discussed below, in the approximate order of the amount of ill health they cause.

Cardiovascular diseases. Hypertension is the commonest cardiovascular disorder: globally 8–18% of adults (300–640 million) have blood pressures of 160/95 mm Hg and above. Cardiovascular diseases cause one-quarter (12 million) of the deaths in the world. In developed countries they are responsible for up to half of all deaths, and in many developing countries they are a leading cause of death. Coronary heart disease has already reached significant dimensions in many developing countries, and there is a need for action to inhibit the spread of associated risk factors (tobacco smoking, hypertension, high serum cholesterol, high alcohol intake, excess weight, and inactivity) in the community.

Rheumatic fever and rheumatic heart disease, though preventable, still affect large numbers of young people in underprivileged communities. In developing countries, these diseases account for more than three out of each ten cardiac cases admitted to hospital.

Over the past two decades, significant declines in cardiovascular disease mortality have been registered in a number of developed countries and these declines have continued in the 1980s. Effective health promotion campaigns targeted at reducing the prevalence of the principal risk factors for these diseases have been an important factor in bringing about these declines.

Chronic respiratory diseases. In the United Kingdom respiratory diseases account for one-quarter of general practitioner consultations. The most prevalent of them, chronic

Fig. 5.7
Estimated global distribution of adult HIV infections – 1991

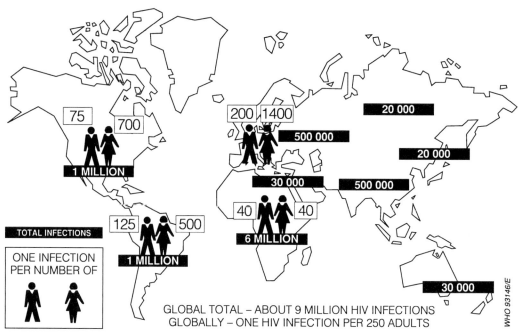

GLOBAL TOTAL – ABOUT 9 MILLION HIV INFECTIONS
GLOBALLY – ONE HIV INFECTION PER 250 ADULTS

The estimated cumulative global total of HIV-infected adults in 1991 is about 9 million, which means that, for the world population, 1 in every 250 adults is infected with HIV. Infection rates vary widely in different regions of the world. The highest rates are in sub-Saharan Africa, where 1 in 40 men and 1 in 40 women are estimated to be infected, with an estimated cumulative total of close to 6 million.

bronchitis, afflicts 8–17% of the adult population. These figures are typical for Europe. Data collected in four African countries among adults aged 20 and over show that 10–20% of them have symptoms of chronic bronchitis. Similar figures were obtained in India and Nepal. The prevalence thus appears to be 300–600 million cases globally. Deaths from chronic obstructive lung disease (basically chronic bronchitis and emphysema) are 385 000 in developed and 2.3 million in developing countries, total 2.7 million deaths worldwide per year. Indoor air pollution is a major cause of these diseases in countries such as China, where brown coal is still widely used for domestic heating and cooking. On the other hand, in countries such as the United States and the United Kingdom, where cigarette smoking has been prevalent for many years, more than 70% of these deaths are attributable to smoking (6).

Recently there has been increasing concern in the developed countries with mortality from asthma. The disease has been investigated as an avoidable cause of death in the European Community and is now used as an indicator of air pollution in the United States.

Diabetes mellitus. This condition is being recognized as an increasingly important problem to the public health of developing and developed countries alike. Unless effective measures are taken the situation will worsen steadily as urbanization and population aging continues, since older people are more susceptible to one form of the disease.

116

It is predicted that one in every five North Americans will develop diabetes by the age of 70 years, and in 1987 the costs relating to diabetes in the United States were US$ 20 billion. In Europe the prevalence is 2–5% in the adult population. Immigrant Indian populations in Fiji, Mauritius, and South Africa all have a prevalence of diabetes of over 10%, rising to approximately 25% by the age of 60 years. There are at least 60 million adult diabetics in the world.

As the epidemic of diabetes develops, the greatest impact is likely to occur in developing countries, both because of the greater genetic susceptibility of their populations to the disease and because of lack of health care facilities to avert its complications. Diabetes is strongly linked with the adoption of a Western lifestyle. As with the other major noncommunicable diseases, the factors most likely to be responsible include obesity, lack of physical exercise, and inappropriate diet. Therefore, diabetes is also potentially preventable.

Cancer. Every year about 7 million new cases occur, half of them in developing countries. Prevalence data indicate that there are currently about 14 million patients with cancer, and about 5 million die of it yearly. In developed countries, two-thirds of male and 60% of female cancer patients will die of their disease; in developing countries, the figures are much higher. Cancer incidence is expected to rise in nearly all parts of the world. The major reasons are a general increase in tobacco use and the progress made against other major health problems, particularly the infectious diseases, which means that people are surviving longer and are hence at greater risk of developing cancer.

Around 70% of cancers are attributable to life style and the environment, and at least one-third ought to be preventable if we act on existing knowledge. The genes responsible for a disposition towards developing stomach and colon cancer have now been identified, opening up the possibility of prevention and eventual genetic treatment.

Much of the rise in cancer can be directly attributed to the massive increase in cigarette smoking which has taken place over the past two or three decades. As a result, lung cancer incidence is increasing in many parts of the world and globally has become the most frequent site of cancer. In some countries, such as the United Kingdom and Finland, successful public health campaigns have led to a marked reduction in smoking prevalence in males at least, with a consequent decline in lung cancer mortality.

Mental and neurological disorders

In the world today there are at least 300 million people suffering from a mental or neurological disorder or impairment that mars their lives and presents a heavy burden for their families and communities.

Societies in almost all parts of the world are characterized by the increasing rapidity of social change, owing in part to fast technological development. This has numerous consequences for mental health and development. For example, occupational or technical skills, highly valued for generations, lose their societal significance, and formerly respected groups find themselves unemployed, underemployed or in a situation where they are no longer considered to be making a contribution to the society in which they live. Numerous demographic factors also contribute to change or are a result of it; the size of the aging population, for example, increases because of increasing life expectancy, the proportion of women employed outside the home increases, and the number of people living in urban areas grows inexorably. High divorce rates and the extraordinarily high number of broken or incomplete families in many countries increase the number of individuals vulnerable to mental, behavioural and psychosocial disorder or environmental maladaptation, and decrease the family's capacity to help a mentally disabled member. The breakdown of the extended family in many developing countries, very often directly linked to economic development, leaves people less well able to cope with new situations or problems.

In terms of amount of suffering, epilepsy affects around 8 million people in developed countries and over 35 million in the rest of the world.

The world population of the mentally retarded numbers between 90 and 130 million. Schizophrenia and other psychoses affect 55 million and some 120 million suffer from affective disorders. The senile dementias affect 5–8% of the population aged over 65, or around 30 million old people. Worldwide, 15–35% of all first-level care consultations are mainly for psychological disorders.

Injuries

This category includes injuries caused by all types of accidents and disasters – burns, drowning, poisoning, and violence. Their causes include unsafe working conditions, inadequate housing, poor road engineering, the widespread use of agricultural and other chemicals without proper precautions, smoking (fires), social breakdown, and military conflicts.

Injuries remain a persistent if not increasing cause of death and disability, particularly in the young, in the majority of countries, both developed and developing. Available figures for mortality from non-intentional injury clearly show that it occupies the first place for childhood (5 years and over), adolescent, and young adult mortality, and when intentional types of injury (homicide) are included they can represent the first cause of mortality for those age-groups combined (Thailand, some Latin American countries).

Other parameters, which have not changed during the period considered, are the high rate for loss of working years of life, and for disabilities caused by brain trauma, and the high economic cost (about US$ 100 billion in the United States per year). For other information on disability, see the next section.

Top of the list of types of accident are traffic accidents. Ironically, the use of seat belts has reduced deaths but increased the amount of disability from such accidents since survivors may be grossly crippled or disfigured. There are also, on average, 90 000 occupational injuries with 400 deaths every day, totalling 32.7 million occupational injuries and 146 000 deaths per year, which leave behind a large residue of people with more or less permanent disabilities. Agrochemicals cause about 4 million poisonings annually, mostly among poorly protected labourers in the developing world.

More accidents occur at home than at work, probably because most of the world's population spends more hours at home than at work. Males are the more vulnerable group for accidents, and the underprivileged are more vulnerable than other socioeconomic groups. The health and economic consequences of falls among the elderly are becoming a matter of concern.

Disability

Not everyone who falls ill or has an accident will be cured, and those who die as a result rarely do so promptly. Progress in methods of care is postponing death in an increasing number of cases. This leads to an increasing number of survivors with some degree of long-term impairment of organs or physical disability, or both, which may prevent them from coping with the demands made by the social or physical environment. Some causes of disability and handicap are increasing in importance, such as the chronic diseases of the lungs induced by smoking or the apocalyptic toll of traffic accidents throughout the world. Increases in longevity lead to an increase in the prevalence of persons with disabilities of varying severity. The proportion of the elderly population in developing countries will increase, and they will add to the existing numbers of those disabled earlier in life by the consequences of malnutrition and diseases such as poliomyelitis and measles.

Information on the extent of disability worldwide is beginning to be collected in a standardized manner based on the categories in WHO's international classification of impairments, disabilities, and handicaps (7). Estimates of the percentage of persons with disabilities vary depending on the types of questions used. Surveys using standardized screening methods show that up to 5% of the population may present disabilities; this percentage is higher where other screening methods have been used (mainly Europe and North America). But the relatively high levels found in developed countries are not solely due to a difference in methods; those countries contain a higher proportion of older people than the others.

Available data generally concentrate on prevalence rather than incidence of disability, and it is not easy to derive information on trends. Rates from diverse national collection sources are not fully comparable at present. However, the relationships found between disability and other demographic or socioeconomic variables are fairly consistent – for instance, it is generally the case that disabilities are more prevalent among the poor.

There are 31 million blind people in the world, more than 90% of them in developing countries. This proportion is tending to increase, as the least developed countries are particularly exposed to public health problems of blinding diseases related to low standards of living, lack of education, and insufficient eye health care services. The main global causes of blindness and their relative importance are well known: cataract around 50%, communicable eye diseases 25%, onchocerciasis and vitamin A deficiency 10%, glaucoma 10%, and other causes (diabetes, trauma etc.) 5%.

The global trend is that cataract is increasing in importance because of its relationship to aging and the growing proportion of elderly people in many populations. Trachoma and other communicable eye diseases are gradually being brought under control in many countries but re-main a serious problem in less developed rural areas and urban slums. Onchocerciasis and vitamin A deficiency (xerophthalmia) are focal diseases in certain areas.

The prevention and control of blindness are related to the coverage provided by health services (ivermectin, vitamin A supplementation, and nutrition education). Glaucoma and diabetes are increasingly important causes of visual loss in developing countries. The priority geographical areas for action to prevent blindness in 1990 stand out quite clearly as Africa and Asia. Technically the enormous challenge is to provide cataract surgery to the approximately 13 million people who need such an operation today.

Oral health

Dental decay is one of the commonest health problems in the western world. The mean number of decayed, missing, and filled teeth at 12 years is perhaps the most informative and widely available indicator of achievement. The global goal is a score of no more than 3 at 12 years of age. Since 1980, improvements in oral health have been registered in a much higher proportion of developed than developing countries; indeed, more of the developing and least developed countries showed a deterioration rather than an improvement.

In the past six years, developing countries have started to recognize the high percentage of the population that has no access to basic or emergency oral health care. There is also a greater awareness that relying on dentists and the use of expensive, sophisticated equipment cannot promote oral health in all areas or ensure equity of essential care. At least 20 developing countries have now started pilot oral health projects in a district or province, with the aim of identifying affordable and sustainable activities to extend care to rural and disadvantaged urban communities.

In the developed countries, dramatic decreases in common oral diseases have continued. Self-care and self-assessment campaigns for the public, developed through collaboration with the profession and industry, have been major forces in maintaining and extending this improvement. A major breakthrough has been the realization that effective retraining and continuing education programmes are essential to ensure the continuing competence of oral health care professionals.

Suicide

Disturbingly, there have been significant increases in suicides in a number of countries. In many countries the suicide rate has risen dramatically since the 1950s, even doubling or tripling in some instances. A large proportion of people committing suicide are found to have high blood levels of alcohol. Much of the increase in suicides has taken place among adolescents and young adults, in whom suicide ranks as a major cause of death (2).

Lifestyle factors affecting health and survival

Introduction

The health of populations is determined by a variety of factors linked to socioeconomic development. In the broadest sense, these factors may be thought of as falling into the following categories: the availability and efficacy of health care, biological factors, the impact of the environment, and personal behaviour and lifestyle. Many aspects of these are discussed elsewhere in this report. This section will therefore concentrate on the lifestyle issues of food and nutrition, tobacco, and the use of alcohol and drugs.

Food, nutrition, and disease

Foodborne diseases, transmitted through consumption of contaminated food and drink, are an increasing health problem all over the world, and in a large majority of cases they are caused by microbes. In developing countries these are responsible for a wide range of diseases (e.g., cholera, salmonellosis, shigellosis, typhoid and paratyphoid fevers, brucellosis, poliomyelitis, and amoebiasis). Diarrhoeal diseases, especially infant diarrhoea, are the dominant problem and indeed one of massive proportions. Formerly, it was thought that contaminated water supplies were the main source of pathogens causing diarrhoea, but now it is believed that up to 70% of diarrhoeal episodes may be due to foodborne agents.

In developed countries, with improvements in standards of personal hygiene, development of basic sanitation, food control infrastructure, and the application of technologies such as pasteurization, many foodborne diseases have been either eliminated or considerably reduced. Nevertheless, some other foodborne diseases such as non-typhoid salmonellosis and campylobacteriosis have increased to such an extent that they have become a serious public health problem. In addition, many of the developed countries are experiencing the emergence of relatively new problems such as listeriosis which affect predominantly the elderly, immunocompromised patients, pregnant women, and neonates.

Besides health problems, food contamination has serious social and economic consequences, especially in countries with limited resources. The economic losses due to foodborne diseases alone can be enormous. These include loss of income, reduced productivity, and higher medical care costs. The cholera epidemic in Peru in 1991 is an example of the impact that food contamination may have on the economy of a country. On the one hand, the country had to sustain the enormous costs inflicted by the medical care of thousands of people affected by the epidemic and, on the other hand, it had to face a substantial decrease in its food exports, as many countries decided to stop or restrict food imports because of presumed food contamination. In addition, the outbreak has also affected the tourist industry, which is a significant source of foreign earnings.

Nutritional status varies markedly within populations, with very significant consequences for health status. Studies throughout the developing world have consistently found that women's calorie intake, and in particular that of pregnant and lactating women, is often well below the minimum daily requirements. As a consequence, poor maternal nutrition in developing countries is a major factor contributing to low birthweight, which in turn exerts a significant influence on child survival (see Fig. 5.8).

According to a recent assessment of children's nutritional levels:

- more than one-third of children under five (150 million) in the developing world, excluding China, are underweight;
- about 163 million children are stunted (below height-for-age) and 35 million are wasted (below weight-for-age);
- more than one in six malnourished children, about 23 million, are severely malnourished (8).

Millions of children suffer from cretinism and other permanent brain damage because their diets and those of their parents are deficient in iodine, or they go blind and even die from lack of vitamin A.

Asia, where nearly one child in two is malnourished, is the most affected region. At least two-thirds of the malnourished children in the world are in Asia, whatever indicator one uses, and almost half of the world's malnourished children live in the eight nations of south Asia. Latin America is the least affected developing region. The prevalence of malnutrition in rural areas is consistently one-and-a-half times greater than that in urban areas.

Enough is now known about proper nutrition to be able to correct the deficiencies that are not due to the sheer lack of enough to eat, and to prevent the development of disorders due to feasting not wisely but too well. In Nepal, a child survival project has taught village mothers, by means of pictures, what foods to give their children to avoid vitamin A deficiency and nutritional blindness. The results have been striking: after only two years, a greater reduction in corneal eye signs was found in those villages than in others that had received megadose vitamin A capsules but no health education. If such an outcome can be achieved by illiterate mothers in one of the least developed countries in the world, how much more, in other areas of nutrition, should be achievable in nations with higher levels of education?

Other encouraging signs are that people in affluent societies are taking more care about what they eat and taking exercise when needed. People with hypertension are controlling their condition by watching their diet, so that they do not progress to heart disease and related problems. Governments, often prodded by consumer associations, are insisting on clear, detailed labelling of the nutritional content of packaged foods and drinks, and banning the use of potentially harmful pesticides, preservatives, and colorants in them. Best of all, on the basis of the latest knowledge of human dietary requirements, more and more countries are adopting national nutrition policies for their people (9).

Tobacco

Currently, tobacco use accounts for 3 million deaths per year, with slightly more than half of these occurring in the developed world where the cumulative exposure (primarily smoking) has been much higher than in the developing world. Over the past decade or so, there have been very significant changes in consumption patterns: cigarette consumption and smoking prevalence have been stagnating or even falling in several developed countries, most notably the United States, Australia, and some west European countries but rising in many developing countries and in eastern Europe, where the situation is quite alarming, especially among men.

In China, for example, which alone accounts for almost one-third of the entire population of the developing world, the consumption of cigarettes increased from 500 billion in 1978 to 1400 billion in 1987: this represents one-quarter of the world's total cigarette consumption. About 6 out of 10 Chinese men smoke, and other surveys conducted during the 1980s indicate that in almost 60% of developing countries surveyed over half of the men smoke, compared with this number in fewer than 30% of developed countries.

In many developed countries, during a period when smoking by men has been falling from its former very high levels, cigarette smoking by women has increased. This appears to be associated with female emancipation and the greater involvement of women in gainful employment. Adolescent girls in these countries are increasingly taking up the habit, and a situation is fast approaching when female smokers will predominate. Another characteristic in developed countries is a higher smoking prevalence at lower socioeconomic levels, among blue-collar workers, disadvantaged groups, and ethnic minorities.

Tobacco chewing, which is as dangerous as smoking in terms of nicotine addiction, is a major cause of oral cancer and a serious health problem in the countries of the Indian subcontinent. It is nowadays less frequently encountered in most developed countries, but attempts to reintroduce it in the form of moist snuff, and thereby instil the habit for further exploitation, particularly among young people, are being made in many countries. On a more positive note, the last few years have been characterized by increasing legislation ensuring the right to a smoke-free environment and limiting the promotion of tobacco products.

Global indicator 8
The percentage of newborns weighing at least 2500 grams at birth, and the percentage of children whose weight-for-age and/or weight-for-height are acceptable.

Fig. 5.8
Birthweight: percentage of newborns weighing at least 2500 grams (global indicator 8.1), 1985 and 1991

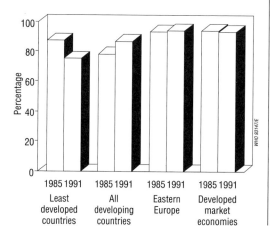

Alcohol and drug abuse

While rates of alcohol consumption and alcohol-related problems are beginning to level off in some developed countries of Europe, the production and consumption of alcohol is increasing in a number of developing countries, particularly in Africa, the Americas, and the western Pacific. Major alcohol-related causes of death include stroke, motor vehicle accidents, liver cirrhosis, suicide, alcohol dependence syndrome, and cancers of the mouth, pharynx, oesophagus, breast, and colon.

It is difficult to quantify the contribution of excess alcohol consumption to mortality without detailed epidemiological studies. In countries where these have been carried out, typically about one-quarter of suicides and 30–35% of road traffic fatalities were attributed to alcohol abuse. In a number of developed countries, an integrated approach to the reduction of alcohol-related problems has been followed with considerable success. In particular, since the early 1970s in a number of developed countries, there has been a dramatic decline in the incidence of fatal traffic accidents involving drivers who had consumed alcohol, which in turn has been a principal factor in the overall reduction in motor vehicle accident deaths during the past decade or so (*10*). The production and consumption of alcohol have continued to increase in many developing countries, in some cases considerably.

In a number of developed countries, an integrated approach to the reduction of alcohol problems has started to have an effect. For example, in Ontario, Canada, the percentage of students who drink alcohol dropped from 75.3% in 1981 to 68.1% in 1987. Traffic accidents involving alcohol-consuming drivers were reduced from about 600 per 100 000 licensed drivers in 1981 to about 300 in 1986.

Drug-related problems are being increasingly reported by national authorities in both developing and developed countries. The abuse of licit drugs is also becoming more common and is now a public health concern in many of the least developed parts of the world, where parallel markets are emerging for the sale of drugs without prescription.

The abuse of injectable drugs such as heroin, cocaine, and amphetamines multiplies health risks, including overdose deaths and the spread of HIV infection. These serious consequences of drug abuse are reported even in countries that were previously unaffected by the problem. Less well recognized but equally significant health problems associated with substance abuse include hepatitis, tuberculosis, cardiovascular diseases, neuropsychiatric disorders, accidents, injuries, violence, suicide, sexually transmitted diseases, and fetal distress and growth problems among children born to drug-abusing mothers. In addition to its direct impact on individual and family health, substance abuse has a major impact on work productivity, family economy, and community organization. The overall costs to society thus go well beyond the immediate health implications.

Globally, there are no estimates of mortality or morbidity due to alcohol and drug abuse but, in the mainly developed countries where such evaluations have been carried out, up to 5% of total mortality has been attributed to alcohol abuse with a further 0.5–1.0% of deaths, mostly of younger adults, due to illicit drug use (*10*).

Summary of trends in health status

The epidemiological transition has continued in developing countries, with cardiovascular disease and cancer rising as a proportion of all deaths even where there has been a decrease in infectious and parasitic diseases.

Tropical diseases seem to have gone on a rampage, with cholera spreading to the Americas for the first time this century, yellow fever and dengue epidemics affecting even greater numbers, the malaria situation deteriorating, schistosomiasis establishing itself in new areas, and leishmaniasis and nonvenereal endemic syphilis increasing. The AIDS pandemic is spreading globally, as also are genital herpes and sexually transmitted chlamydial disease. Pulmonary tuberculosis is on the increase, partly stimulated by HIV co-infection. Pneumonia and hepatitis B remain serious threats. The whole category of chronic noncommunicable disease is increasing, especially in the developing world, where the number of cancer cases has overtaken that in the developed countries. Lung cancer has overtaken breast cancer as the leading cancer in females in some developed countries owing to the spread of the smoking epidemic among women.

Diabetes is increasing everywhere, blindness (especially cataract) is more common, alcohol-related diseases are up (especially in developing countries), as are mental problems and suicide (particularly in the developed countries).

On the other hand some vaccine-preventable diseases of childhood – measles, acute paralytic poliomyelitis, pertussis, and neonatal tetanus – are going down owing to a rapid increase in coverage by immunization programmes. Cardiovascular diseases in developed countries (except eastern Europe) are on the wane owing to the spread of health education, and lung cancer has peaked in males in some developed countries since they began to give up smoking.

In spite of the increase in many diseases and health problems, the overall death rate and the infant and child mortality rates have continued to decrease globally, with a few exceptions in war-torn least developed countries, and life expectancy has continued to increase, except in males in some east European countries. This overall progress largely reflects the major gains made against the vaccine-preventable diseases of early childhood and the deferment of death from some of the major chronic diseases to progressively older ages.

References

1. Sullivan, J. Recent trends in infant and child mortality. In: *World Conference on Demographic and Health Surveys, Washington, DC, 5-7 August 1991* (unpublished).
2. Blum, R.W. Global trends in adolescent health. *Journal of the American Medical Association*, **265** (20): 2176 (1991).
3. Lopez, A.D. & Ruzicka, T. *Sex differentials in mortality trends, determinants and consequences.* Canberra, The Australian University, Department of Demography, 1983.
4. Lopez, A.D. Causes of death: an assessment of global patterns of mortality around 1985. *World health statistics quarterly*, **43** (2): 91–104 (1990).
5. *Current and future dimensions of the HIV/AIDS pandemic.* Geneva, World Health Organization, 1991.
6. US Surgeon General. *Reducing the health consequences of smoking – 25 years of progress.* Rockville, MD, US Department of Health and Human Services, 1989.
7. *International classification of impairments, disabilities and handicaps: a manual of classification relating to the consequences of disease.* Geneva, World Health Organization, 1980.
8. Carlson, B.A. & Wardlaw, T.M. *An assessment of child malnutrition.* New York, United Nations Children's Fund, 1990.
9. *World health*, July–August 1991.
10. Holman, C.D.J. et al. *The quantification of drug-caused morbidity and mortality in Australia.* Canberra, Commonwealth Department of Community Services and Health, 1988.

CHAPTER 6

Health and environment

Introduction

Safe water and basic sanitation have been recognized for centuries as major determinants of health. However, only in 1980 was the first major global initiative taken in the form of the International Drinking Water Supply and Sanitation Decade that mobilized international support and resources to support countries in achieving universal access to safe water and basic sanitation. There has also been an increasing recognition that the maintenance of life on this planet rests on a delicate balance of forces, which is now threatened by the growth of the human population and its increasing exploitation of limited natural resources, leading to pollution of air, water and land. Concern about deforestation, desertification, depletion of the ozone layer, and climatic change has drawn attention to the health implications of environmental problems of a global nature (1). In addition to this broad range of issues are the concerns related to the health impacts of rapid urbanization.

Access to water supply and sanitation

The health burden of unsafe and insufficient quantities of water and inadequate sanitation facilities continues to be borne in terms of high rates of water-related diseases, especially diarrhoeal diseases, schistosomiasis, dracunculiasis, and trachoma. It is often overlooked that the fetching and carrying of water – whether from the village stand-pipe or well or from a source much further away – can consume up to 25% of daytime human energy. The responsibility is usually borne by women and young children, who are often the least nourished and the least healthy members of the family. Moreover, the time required for such tasks often takes several hours - perhaps even a major portion of the day in areas where water is scarce – and may result in poor school attendance.

Hidden in the global figures are huge variations, which mean that, even where coverage has improved significantly, many inhabitants still lack water and sanitation facilities. They frequently have to buy water from private vendors, paying the full market price for water that is often unsafe. Often, the price of water sold by these private vendors is 10 or 20 times the rate paid by residents with a piped water supply. Unaccounted-for water losses, resulting from leakages in taps and mains and from illegal connections, represent more than 50% of the water produced by some cities in developing countries.

The year 1990 marked the conclusion of the highly publicized International Drinking Water Supply and Sanitation Decade (1981–1990). The period 1985–1990 marked however a slow but progressive reduction in the inequities in water supply and sanitation services existing within regions and countries and between urban and rural populations. By 1990, safe water supplies had been extended to 81% of urban dwellers and 58% of rural inhabitants (Fig. 6.1).

125

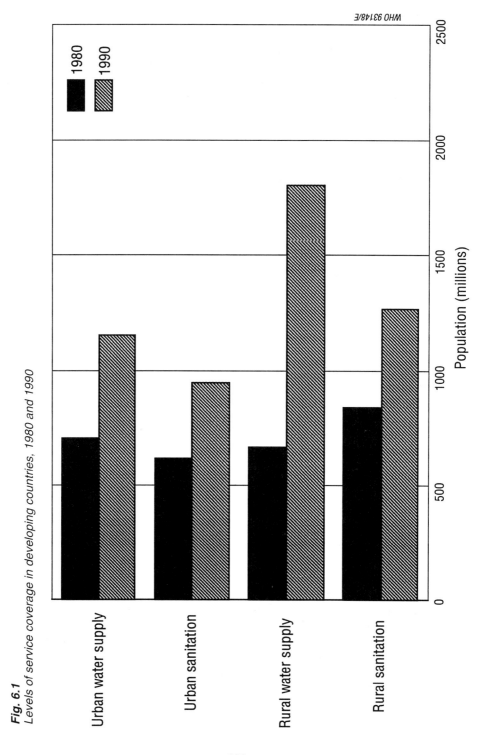

Fig. 6.1
Levels of service coverage in developing countries, 1980 and 1990

Similarly, the 1990 figures for adequate sanitation show a coverage rate of 71% in urban areas and 48% in rural areas. These figures reflect that the emphasis during the Decade was more on the extension of rural water supplies than on urban water supplies, and more on extending water supplies than on adequate sanitation, whether in rural or in urban areas. Despite these increases in the percentage of people supplied with safe water and adequate sanitation, growing numbers of people still remain without access to these basic services because of population increase. In terms of total expenditures for water supply and sanitation, great inequities continue to exist between urban and rural areas. It has been estimated that approximately 80% of all water supply and sanitation investments are devoted to high-cost urban services and only 20% to low-cost rural facilities.

There are many factors that contribute to the lack of progress in countries and to the deterioration of existing water and sanitation facilities. For example, there has been prolonged drought in the Sahelian regions of Africa, while floods and earthquakes have struck Asia. Civil and military strife, poor organizational and management structures, and weak or nonexistent legal frameworks all contribute to this grim scenario. When aid is tied to specific makes and brands of equipment and when insufficient funds are available, the nature of system developed is affected, as well as the ability to maintain it. Systems are often poorly operated and maintained, and this is aggravated by the lack of spare parts, the lack of trained and motivated staff, and the lack of consumer involvement. Weak political commitment at the highest level can be a major additional impediment to making water and sanitation services available. In addition, the worldwide economic recession that began in the early 1980s had a marked effect on the developing countries and inhibited the acceleration of improvements in water supply and sanitation facilities during the latter half of the Decade.

The maintenance of water supplies and sanitation in developing countries, particularly in the rural areas, has been badly neglected. Many systems have fallen into disrepair. In some areas, where water supply is provided primarily through point sources fitted with handpumps, up to 60% of facilities are estimated to be out of order, often because of the unavailability of very simple spare parts such as washers. In some places, however, even when resources were scarce and the situation very difficult, improvements have been made by communities deciding what they needed, participating in the financing, and taking over some of the management responsibilities themselves. For example, a large squatter colony in Orangi Township in Karachi (Pakistan) financed and constructed an underground sewerage system with technical advice and support from outside experts. The system continues to be operated and maintained by the township residents. Three things were essential to the programme's success: community participation; the modification of standard engineering technology and procedures to make them suitable for the community; and redefinition of the working relationships between the community and local government officials.

Several favourable trends begun early in the Decade have continued and gained strength with the passage of time. One trend is that the provision of water for personal hygiene is now considered just as important as safe water for drinking and cooking. In addition to focusing on water supply, overall environmental improvement efforts were expanded to include water quality, sanitation, hygiene education, and general community involvement in local environmental management.

By 1990, a total of 122 countries were cooperating with WHO on the periodic monitoring of their water supply and sanitation progress, a notable advance over the 1985 situation in monitoring coverage at the national level. In achieving the primary goal of expanding water supply and sanitation services to unserved and poorly served communities, greater emphasis is now placed on community-level institutions and on stronger linkages with other health-related programmes, including water-resources management. Hygiene education, community participation, and women's involvement in community decision-making are three key areas important for the sustainability of water supply and sanitation systems. Many countries have carried out training activities and/or formulated appropriate guidelines and curricula for human resources development in water supply and sanitation. The "dual focus" approach, which recognizes the close relationship between improvements in the training of personnel and the enhancement of water supply and sanitation services (given the availability of appropriate resources), has been followed by several countries, including Jordan and the United Republic of Tanzania.

There is now a global acceptance that the eradication of dracunculiasis is possible through improved water supplies. Major national efforts in such countries as Ghana, India, and Nigeria give great promise that this disease can be eradicated during the 1990s. Schistosomiasis has also received increasing attention, especially since recent studies have shown that populations with improved water supplies can have up to 40% lower incidence of the disease than those without. Public water taps alone have been shown to reduce *Schistosoma mansoni* infections by about 20%. Health problems directly resulting from planning procedures that ignored the health effects of water-resources development have occurred over the past five years, such as outbreaks of Japanese encephalitis in the Mahaweli irrigation project (Sri Lanka) in 1987–1988, and a dramatic rise in the prevalence of schistosomiasis in Senegal following the construction of the Diama Dam. In several countries steps have been taken towards the creation of intersectoral bodies to deal with these problems, but such structures prove remarkably ephemeral in times of political instability.

Availability of water

In focusing on access to safe water, one should not forget the importance of the *availability* of water. Recently concerns over the quantity and quality of fresh water resources have been emerging as many countries are suffering from the effects of pollution of their waters, aggravated by drought, depletion of aquifers, and deforestation. The availability of fresh-water resources per capita varies widely; many areas of the world are semi-arid, with highly variable rainfall and recurrent droughts. North and sub-Saharan Africa, the Arabian Peninsula, southern Iran, Pakistan, and western India, for example, suffer from rainfall variability. In the Sahel, the rainfall is not only unreliable but is less now than it was 30 years ago. In Asia, water supply per capita is less than half the global average, and the continent's run-off is the least stable of all the major land masses. In Africa, there is less run-off than the global average, but the main problem is the underdevelopment of water resources in relation to the needs and potential. Overall it appears that about 50 developing countries are approaching a situation of severe scarcity of water. The contamination of water supplies is also posing health risks and is drastically increasing the cost of water-treatment facilities. Polluted inland water and seas are reducing the productivity of fisheries and increasing the health risks of eating fish caught in those waters. Polluted irrigation water poses health risks, undermines long-term crop productivity, and degrades the recreational use and aesthetic aspects of surface water. Surface and ground water sources are being increasingly contaminated in many areas in both developed and developing countries by fertilizers, herbicides, and pesticides used in agriculture, by industrial and residential waste, and by seepage from waste storage and disposal sites. Concern has increased in many countries over the protection and national management of coastal water and marine resources.

Fresh water is limited in quantity, and its

quality has been deteriorating. It is necessary to find new ways of conserving water and implementing existing methods more efficiently and extensively. As new water supplies are developed, account should be taken of the likely adverse impact on the environment. Conserving water and increasing the efficiency of use of household and community water would reduce the need for new plant, water mains, and sewwers – and also cut other associated costs of providing and disposing of water supplies. Efficiency is being increased by reducing losses in the distribution system, as in Brazil, Colombia, and Malaysia, and by using more efficient household fixtures and appliances. It can also be improved through the adoption of better designs for the collection, treatment, and use of domestic waste water for agricultural purposes, as is being done in Chile and Israel. Several technically feasible and economically viable new options are available and could be exploited to improve the availability of fresh water. For example, waste water can be re-used for non-potable purposes, and water used for industrial purposes can be recycled.

Environmental health hazards

Modern synthetic chemicals have become an essential part of human life, sustaining economic activities, increasing agricultural productivity, preventing and controlling diseases, and bringing significant benefits to society. The global health situation is therefore likely to have been improved by their use, but the need to apply appropriate safeguards against their deleterious health effects is indisputable.

Acute and chronic exposures to chemicals from the production, storage, transport, and use of chemicals as well as from accidental discharge are staggering (see Table 6.1). A number of dramatic poisoning episodes, such as the mineral oil poisoning in Spain and the Bhopal catastrophe in India, have made worldwide headlines, but it is likely that the many smaller inci-

dents with workplace chemicals and the use of chemicals or pesticides in the home and in agriculture and vector control create a much larger number of poisonings. For example, agrochemicals alone lead to about 4 million poisonings each year.

Millions of people are exposed to toxic chemicals in food, drinking-water, or air. Naturally occurring toxic chemicals are of particular concern in poor communities with a traditional life style, especially if people get most of their food and all their drinking-water from local sources. Geochemical conditions may create particularly high concentrations of trace elements in food or water, leading to local endemic diseases, which may affect millions of people. Examples include skeletal fluorosis in India, Kaschin-Beck disease in China, and endemic arsenic poisoning in parts of South America. The exact number of people affected by these chemical-related diseases is not known, but indications are that the number is being reduced by the increased awareness of the problems and the prompt action by the countries concerned.

Epidemics of poisoning through naturally occurring toxins such as pyrrolizidine alkaloids in grain have occurred in India and Afghanistan; lathyrism from natural poisons in a local variety of bean occurs in parts of India; poisoning from natural toxins in fish and molluscs is endemic in certain tropical countries; and aflatoxin (a mycotoxin) in peanuts and other foodstuffs is a major problem in parts of Africa and Asia. Again, the total extent of the health impact is unknown, but more and more is learned about local situations as national chemical safety programmes are formulated.

During the past five years, major progress has been achieved in national efforts to identify, prevent, and manage health problems associated with chemical exposure. National chemical safety programmes have been developed in a number of countries in Europe, the Americas, Asia, and the Pacific. These national programmes have included efforts to stimulate

Table 6.1
Extent of human exposure to neurotoxic chemicals, latest available estimate

Chemical	Extent of exposure and numbers affected
Pesticides	
Worldwide	At least 15 000 deaths; more than 1 million cases of poisoning
United States	4–5 million workers exposed; about 300 000 cases of poisoning a year
Honduras	32% of 1100 farmers examined in a study had a decrease in cholinesterase levels in excess of 25%
Cuba	17 500 workers exposed
Organic solvents	
Federal Republic of Germany	1–2 million workers exposed
United States	9.8 million workers exposed
Venezuela	7000 workers exposed
Lead	
United States	12.5 million children at risk from lead exposure
Venezuela	13 760 workers exposed
China	1.7% prevalence of chronic poisoning in 355 000 workers examined

changes in legislation, standards, field-work support, and training in all aspects of chemical safety and to encourage better coordination among the different government sectors concerned.

National training courses were held in a large number of countries, including Canada, Uruguay, and Zimbabwe. They covered general chemical safety or risk assessment; epidemiology as applied to chemical safety; and the control of poisonings. Many developed countries have adequate infrastructures and established mechanisms to respond to chemical emergencies while special poison control centres have been established in several developing countries.

In 1990, the main environmental hazards of concern were still the same as they were in 1985: urban air pollution, indoor air pollution, agrochemicals, the contamination of fresh water and drinking-water supplies, hazardous wastes, and ionizing radiation. There are, of course, others such as noise and non-ionizing radiation that can affect health adversely. New concerns include a possible increase of skin cancer and other diseases as a result of increasing ultraviolet B radiation resulting from depletion of the stratospheric ozone layer.

As regards urban air pollution, the most recent statistics show that an estimated 600 million people live in cities where sulfur dioxide levels exceed WHO health guidelines and 1200 million live in cities where particulate matter exceeds WHO health guidelines (Table 6.2) (2). Most of these cities are in developing countries.

A number of successful actions to control air pollution have been taken at country or local level. Most European countries have made lead-free petrol available and require catalytic converters on all new cars. This will significantly reduce urban air pollution in these countries. Similar measures are being implemented in developing countries, including the Republic of Korea. Car-free days have been instituted in Mexico City, and car-tolls have been used for many years in a number of countries with the aim of reducing air pollution and traffic congestion. However, effective pollution control equipment for industrial sources is out of reach for most developing countries, and polluting industries are frequently exported to these countries without adequate safeguards.

Table 6.2
Estimates of populations residing in urban areas of given air quality

Air quality conditions (annual average)	Number of people (millions)	
	Sulfur dioxide	Suspended particles
Acceptable	625 (35%)	350 (20%)
Marginal	550 (30%)	200 (10%)
Unacceptable	625 (35%)	1250 (70%)

Source: Reference (2)

The major concern for indoor air quality is due to cooking and heating with biomass fuels in several developing countries. The concentrations of many air pollutants inside dwellings are extremely high and may affect as many as 500 million people worldwide. The most important effects are lung and heart diseases.

The degree to which the world's population is exposed to hazardous wastes is not known, but in certain regions it could be substantial. The effects include accidental injuries resulting from improper handling of chemical wastes, acute poisoning (in particular in people who make their living from scavenging dumps and disposal sites), chronic poisoning caused by long-term exposure to chemicals present in air, water, and food, and the spread of infectious and parasitic diseases from hospital wastes, sewage, and sewage sludge. Certain hazards such as mercury in wastes from gold mining in Brazil and the Philippines have received particular attention.

While exposure to ionizing radiation in industry is well controlled all over the world, accidental releases are of major concern. There was still in 1990 the great problem of the long-term health consequences for the people in the areas affected by the accident at the Chernobyl nuclear power plant. The consequences of such accidents are being investigated through international initiatives such as the WHO international programme on the health effects of the Chernobyl accident.

There has been a major increase in political awareness of environmental pollution and its effects on the environment and health. Between 1985 and 1990 this awareness reached the highest political levels and has led to much increased activity on various global environmental issues ranging from acid rain and the depletion of the ozone layer to transboundary movement of hazardous wastes and global warming. This increased awareness has also "spilled over" into other fields. As a result, more positive action to safeguard the environment is being envisaged.

In spite of increased awareness, national capabilities in 1989 for environmental pollution control seemed to have improved very little since 1984. Most developing countries are still grossly deficient in environmental protection. Even the majority of the developed countries are far from having adequate facilities and capabilities for dealing with the problems at hand.

It should be noted that not all the environmental problems were dealt with to the same degree by national programmes. Drinking-water quality and water pollution in general received much more attention than air pollution, solid waste, or noise. The basic problem is still lack of resources, both funds and of manpower. Though increased awareness has often led to adequate legislation and regulations, the implementation of the law has been poor. In some cases a total lack of monitoring or enforcement has rendered the legislation and regulations meaningless. There is an overall recognition of this problem. Increasing emphasis has been placed on human resource development and applied research. Professional training programmes at national level have also improved the awareness of policy-makers and planners in this area in many countries (Table 6.3).

Table 6.3
Changes in indicator scores relating to environmental activities, 1984 and 1989

Indicator	1984 Index	1989 Index
Legislation in place	1.53	1.63
Strategy formulated	1.12	1.19
Standards set	1.39	1.68
Assessment of laboratories	1.53	1.73
Enforcement and monitoring	1.31	1.46
Staffing adequacy	1.53	1.53
Research and forecasting	1.45	1.55
Intersectoral coordination	1.22	1.53
Health authority involved	1.56	1.61
Vertical delegation	1.58	1.58

Source: *Combating environmental pollution; national capabilities for health protection.* Geneva, World Health Organization, 1991 (document WHO/PEP/91.14).

Environmental health services inside the public health structures still need strengthening, at both national and local level. However, progress has been reported in Mediterranean countries, eastern Asian countries, and several African countries, where environmental health units are incorporated into health ministries. Training institutions for environmental health personnel have continued to develop in low-income countries, but this development is limited by the lack of resources to hire environmental health graduates.

Housing and health

Continued rapid population growth and the pervasive spread of poverty, particularly in developing countries, are placing a strain on society's capacity to provide housing and neighbourhood environmental health services. In many developing countries the degradation of living conditions is of crisis proportions. A massive growth in urban populations has taken place without the development of adequate housing, infrastructure, and employment. In both urban and rural areas, a large burden of disease and premature death is caused by deficiencies in housing and in basic health and environmental services.

A WHO survey carried out in 1987 showed that few of the countries to be surveyed were actively responding to the problems of poor housing and environmental conditions in human settlements and that even when they did respond it was mainly the urban population that was targeted (3). Awareness and responsiveness to the health problems associated with inadequate and poor-quality housing and rapid urban growth are increasing generally, as is the need to improve the capacity of municipal governments. City networking approaches, encompassing technology exchange, community participation, and "enabling policies" of municipal governments (to support self-reliant action by community members in improving environmental conditions in their own neighbourhoods), have been developed and implemented to improve urban environmental health. Usually, economic development was given preference over social development, and the satisfaction of other social needs was given preference over improvements in housing. Community organizations for ensuring a healthy environment were weak or absent in about two-thirds of countries and where they existed, they were mainly in rural areas. They were weakest among disadvantaged populations. Remedial programmes for people in disadvantaged housing settings were rare, and where they existed they were mainly directed to urban slums, to the neglect of migrant and nomadic populations. In most of the countries, the effectiveness of mechanisms for intersectoral action was minimal or totally lacking, especially in rural settings. While standards for urban housing were being set, little was being done for rural housing. Ministries of health exercised some influence in government decisions on housing development, but in general, provision of medical care and disease-prevention activities took precedence over environmental health improvements. Most countries, particularly the less developed ones, were inhibited by lack of information from participating effectively in health advocacy or technical support. More attention was paid to health aspects such as the siting and conditions of housing when human settlements were being planned.

Management of environmental resources (4,5)

Natural disasters such as earthquakes, windstorms, tsunamis, floods and landslides, volcanic eruption, and forest fires are estimated to have claimed more than 3 million lives worldwide in the past two decades, affected the lives of about 800 million people and caused irreversible damage exceeding US$ 25 billion. Owing to the neglect of the environment, disasters are likely to occur more frequently and possibly with greater intensity. Health also depends on a good environment where people are protected from physical, chemical, and biological hazards and where the resources essential to health are protected – including soil, water, and plants and the natural cycle on which they depend. However, we are increasingly facing the question of limited environmental space and, as Robert Heilbroner called it, "the closing window of environmental tolerance" (6). The environmental basis for health is being undermined by increasing resource use, the generation of more wastes, and population growth. Debates about development and the elimination of poverty have given little attention to health, except to assume that increasing levels of production to raise personal and national income would bring better health. There has been little recognition that human health and well-being depend on the continued

availability of environmental resources such as clean air, safe water, productive land, and the safe disposal of domestic, industrial, and agricultural wastes without exposing people to pathogens and toxic substances. Initiatives have been taken to formulate and implement measures to safeguard environmental services and to keep the earth habitable.

Sustainability of the development process demands changes in current patterns of growth that are less resource- and energy-intensive and more equitable. Many environmental risks stemming from economic activities cross national boundaries and some are global in scope. The risks of harmful effects from hazardous wastes and from an increasing concentration of carbon dioxide and other greenhouse gases in the atmosphere, though mainly stemming from economic activities in the developed countries, are shared by all countries whether they benefit from these activities or not. This section reviews some of these issues of global concern, since action has to be initiated now or accelerated if we are to avoid irreversible losses of potentially renewable resources (7).

Loss of biodiversity

As a result of human encroachment on hitherto undeveloped or uninhabited land areas and of ecosystem change, the world's diversity of species and the habitats in which they live are decreasing rapidly. As estimates of the total number of plant and animal species vary from 10 to 80 million, it is impossible to quantify the loss of biodiversity in absolute terms. It is believed however, that losses of tropical rainforest species alone may amount to 0.2–0.3% per year, or 100 species per day. The effects of these losses on human health are most directly felt in the declining availability of medicinal plant species, of which thousands are expected to disappear before the year 2000. Ancestral strains of human food crops and domesticated animals will also be affected, as well as biological control agents used to combat agricultural pests and human and animal diseases. Efforts are being made to mobilize political support for a Global Biodiversity Convention, which is proposed for adoption at the United Nations Conference on Environment and Development in 1992.

Deforestation

On a global basis, the world's forests are disappearing at a rate of 15 million hectares each year with most of the losses occurring in the humid parts of Africa, Asia, and Latin America. Deforestation is not caused simply by population; it is also due to timber extraction for foreign exchange, clearance for agricultural purposes, and encroachment by landless peasants. To alleviate tropical deforestation and promote sustainable exploitation of the world's forests, countries have been increasingly assessing the value of their forest resources in a comprehensive way. Multipurpose forest management involving the production of timber, non-wood forest products, fuel wood, and fodder, together with wildlife management and watershed management, is being taken seriously, and the 1985 initiative – the Tropical Forestry Action Plan – to coordinate human needs, environment management, and sustainable forest development, has been slowly gaining recognition by concerned countries.

Desertification and soil degradation

Desertification is increasingly becoming a worldwide threat affecting more than a hundred countries. About 850 million people live on 35% of the earth's surface consisting of arid, semi-arid, and sub-humid zones, all at risk of desertification. Desertification worldwide is proceeding at about 6 million hectares a year, and owing to soil erosion an additional 20 million hectares of agricultural land have become barren. Two-fifths of Africa's non-desert land risks being turned to desert, as does one-third of Asia's and one-fifth of Latin America's. About

470 million people are moderately affected and about 190 million are severely affected. The consequences of desertification include increased hunger and death, as well as social instability and conflict when dry land degradation drives ecological refugees in their millions to the cities and across national boundaries. A change in mammalian fauna and arthropods may result in a rise of rodent- and insect-borne diseases. In Africa, for example, the population in agriculture has increased by 2.5–3.0% per year, in pastoral activities by 1.5–2.5% per year and the livestock population from 295 million in 1950 to 521 million in 1983. The combined effects of human and animal pressure on land accelerate environmental degradation, setting in train a process of decreased water infiltration, increased surface run-off, drying up of surface-water resources, and loss of topsoil and soil nutrients.

The substitution of traditional mixed cropping – which includes plants or shrubs along with food crops - by monoculture and poor management of land and water has caused soil erosion and degradation. Although irrigation has greatly improved farm productivity, inappropriate irrigation has wasted water, polluted groundwater and damaged the productivity of millions of hectares. While people are the main agents of desertification, they are also the victims of such desertification, as for example in the 1984–1985 crisis in the Sahel region of Africa.

Greenhouse gases and global warming

Part of the solar radiation falling on the earth's surface is reradiated back at a longer wavelength and is partially absorbed by gases in the atmosphere. This absorption of energy raises the temperature of the atmosphere and constitutes the "greenhouse effect".

The primary greenhouse gases of concern are carbon dioxide, chlorofluorocarbons, halons, methane, nitrous oxide, and ozone. These contribute directly to the greenhouse effect through their thermodynamic properties. There are other gases that, while not having a direct thermal effect, contribute indirectly through their chemical reactions with the greenhouse gases, thus affecting the concentrations of the latter. Examples of such gases are nitric oxide and carbon monoxide. Some of the greenhouse gases, such as ozone and methane, have both direct and indirect effects.

Emissions of greenhouse gases into the atmosphere have been increasing ever since the beginning of the industrial revolution. Today the levels are such that, if continued over the next decades, they could lead to a rise in mean global temperature greater than any experienced in human history. Besides the changes in global climate and climate distribution that this would include, the global environment would also be affected by an increase in ultraviolet radiation owing to a decrease in stratospheric ozone caused by the accumulation of chlorofluorocarbons and other man-made compounds in the

atmosphere. A major component of emissions of carbon dioxide is from the combustion of fossil fuels. While the climatic changes that might be produced are difficult to predict, it is generally conceded that the main effects would include an increase of about 3°C in the average global surface temperature by the year 2030, a rise in sea level of 0.1–0.3 metres by 2050, and an increase in the occurrence of extreme climatic events such as cyclones, heatwaves, and droughts.

A direct health effect of global warming in the form of heatwaves will adversely affect individuals with failing functions of the cardiovascular, respiratory, renal, endocrine, or immune systems, as well as those with immature or reduced adaptive regulatory functions such as infants and the elderly. Indirect effects on health might include a change in the distribution of some vector-borne diseases such as malaria and dengue (Table 6.4), the migration of refugees following an increase in natural disasters such as flooding, malnutrition following a loss of

Table 6.4
Global status of major vector-borne diseases and likelihood of change with climate, around 1989

	Population at risk[a] (millions)	Prevalence of infection (millions)	Present distribution	Possible change of distribution as a result of climatic change[b]
Malaria	2100	270	tropics/subtropics	+++
Lymphatic filariases	900	90.2	tropics/subtropics	+
Onchocerciasis	90	17.8	Africa/Latin America	+
Schistosomiasis	600	200	tropics/subtropics	++
African trypanosomiasis	50	[c]	tropical Africa	+
Leishmaniases	350	12[d]	Asia/southern Europe/Africa/ South America	?
Dracunculiasis	63	1	tropics (Africa/Asia)	o
Dengue			tropics/subtropics	++
Yellow fever	No estimates available		Africa/Latin America	+
Japanese encephalitis	–,,–		Eastern Asia	+
Other arboviral disease	–,,–		—	+

[a] Based on a world population estimated at 4800 million in 1989.
[b] o = unlikely; + = likely; ++ = very likely; +++ = extremely likely; ? = not known.
[c] Incidence of 25 000 new cases per year.
[d] Incidence of 400 000 new cases per year.

marginal crops due to climate change, and an increase in waterborne diseases due to contamination of water supplies (8).

In view of the likelihood of a future climatic change of possibly catastrophic impact, several international initiatives have already been started. A major report of the Intergovernmental Panel on Climate Change in June 1990 emphasized the potential gravity of the effects of climate change. The Intergovernmental Negotiating Committee for a Framework Convention on Climate Change is currently working towards a consensus commitment on measures to counter the effects of climate change.

Depletion of the ozone layer

Over the past 20 years, recorded measurements have disclosed a significant decrease in stratospheric ozone concentrations, especially in the northern hemisphere. This reduction is brought about by a reaction between the ozone and several chemicals, largely chlorofluorocarbons and halons, and can result in an increase in biologically active ultraviolet radiation reaching the earth's surface. This is because ozone mainly absorbs ultraviolet with wavelengths less than 325 nm.

The health effects of ultraviolet radiation that might be expected include an increase in non-melanoma skin cancer as well as malignant melanoma; an increase in eye diseases, largely cataract; and a possible reduction in the immune response. Marine organisms in the upper layers of the sea may be endangered by an increase in ultraviolet radiation, which damages various aquatic larvae and decreases the production of algae. While the effect on terrestrial plants is variable, some sensitive species often display reductions in growth (plant height, dry weight, leaf area, etc.), photosynthetic activity, and flowering. This could affect vulnerable agricultural crops (8).

International efforts to combat the destruction of the ozone layer began with the signing of the Vienna Convention for the Protection of the Ozone Layer in March 1985. At the time of writing, 76 states and the European Economic Community have become Parties to the Convention. Within the framework of this Convention, 70 states and the EEC have become Parties to the Montreal Protocol on Substances that Deplete the Ozone Layer, which entered into force in January 1989.

Transboundary air pollution

Gaseous pollution of the atmosphere also includes the formation of sulfur and nitrogen oxides from energy production, industrial processes, and motor vehicles. In addition to their potential direct effects on human health, these emissions are responsible for the atmospheric formation of acid aerosols, which result in both dry and wet acid deposition. This phenomenon is prevalent in several regions of the world, including much of Europe, eastern North America, China, and parts of south-east Asia and Latin America. It is known that acid deposition has adverse effects on freshwater aquatic ecosystems, vegetation, and the built environment, but there could also be indirect effects on human health. Acidification of water and soils can mobilize certain heavy metals. For example, in an acidified environment, mercury may be mobilized and accumulate in freshwater fish, which in turn may be consumed. Acidification of drinking-water may also increase the mobilization of metals such as lead, which is used in water pipes, contaminating water supplies. Concentrations of aluminium in drinking-water may also be enhanced by acidification. Initial steps such as the EEC Protocol have been taken to promote preventive measures internationally.

Conclusion

Awareness of environmental problems by politicians and the public alike has increased worldwide owing, in particular, to the much publicized phenomena of a global or regional nature that pose a threat to human health and the environment, including the depletion of the protective stratospheric ozone layer, the predicted global climate change, and the transboundary movement of hazardous wastes. Regrettably, this increase in general awareness has, in the first instance, focused on associated environmental impacts rather than the consequences to human health.

Owing to an increasing socioeconomic imbalance between developing and developed countries, traditional environmental health concerns related to uncontrolled urbanization and inadequate water supplies and sanitation facilities have not decreased during the reporting period. In fact, this imbalance has led to an increase in poverty and population growth, in particular in cities of the developing world, which are already bursting at the seams. Population growth is widely outpacing the rate at which water supply and sanitation facilities and adequate housing are provided. In addition, health impacts from unsafe food and drinking-water supplies, air pollution outdoors and indoors, and the inappropriate use of chemicals in agriculture, are still a leading cause of suffering and death.

However, global efforts are now being initiated to create an economic environment in which it is more profitable to conserve resources than destroy them. Countries in both the developing and developed world have started action to reduce environmental degradation and to restore the resource base through legislation, regulation, and the application of better technology.

A major international initiative was launched to this end by the United Nations General Assembly in 1989 by adopting resolution 44/228, which calls for the convening of a United Nations Conference on Environment and Development in 1992. This conference may be considered as a milestone in the international efforts to agree on a sustainable course of development by adopting Agenda 21, an action programme for the twenty-first century. The health sector has to be fully involved in shaping this action programme, building on the increased efforts to put health plainly on the environment and development agenda in the future. A profound analysis of health determinants in the context of environment and development was provided to the conference through the WHO Commission on Health and Environment (established in 1990); it is expected that significant initiatives will be launched following this conference to promote and protect health in the face of the environmental and developmental crisis.

References

1. *1989 report on the world social situation.* New York, United Nations, 1989.
2. *Global pollution and health.* London, United Nations Environment Programme/World Health Organization, 1987.
3. *National capacities and needs in aspects of environmental health in rural and urban development and housing.* Geneva, World Health Organization, 1988 (document WHO/EHE/RUD/88.1).
4. *Environmental data report.* London, United Nations Environment Programme, 1989.
5. *Global outlook 2000.* New York, United Nations, 1990.
6. Heilbroner, R. Reflections (after communism). *The New Yorker*, September 1990.
7. *Development cooperation.* Paris, Organization for Economic Co-operation and Development, 1990.
8. *Potential health effects of climatic change.* Geneva, World Health Organization, 1990 (Report of a WHO task group, document WHO/PEP/90.10).

CHAPTER 7

Assessment of achievements

The Thirty-fourth World Health Assembly in 1981 adopted the Global Strategy for Health for All by the Year 2000 (*1*), which stated that "as a minimum *all* people in *all* countries should have *at least* such a level of health that they are capable of working productively and of participating actively in the social life of the community in which they live". Yet "it was recognized that while different countries will strive to improve the health of their people in keeping with their social and economic capacities, there is a baseline below which no individuals in any country should find themselves". Moreover "to attain such a level of health every individual should have access to primary health care and through it to all levels of a comprehensive health system". The strategy included global targets and a list of indicators to be used for monitoring and evaluation. Minimum (or baseline) values were also incorporated in some of the targets and indicators.

Previous chapters have analysed the status and progress in the implementation of the global strategy and the factors that influenced or constrained this progress. This chapter brings together these findings and presents conclusions on what has been achieved so far in implementing the strategy.

The degree to which the primary health care approach has been adapted and applied when developing national health systems will also be assessed, with particular regard to the main characteristics (essential care, community involvement, appropriate technology and inter-

sectoral cooperation). The framework used here to this end is shown in Fig. 7.1. It should be noted that progress in implementing the global strategy was assessed on three occasions: (i) the first monitoring in 1983; (ii) the first evaluation in 1985; and (iii) the second monitoring in 1988. The present evaluation assesses the achievements in terms of direction and trends during the ten years since 1980, using the global targets and indicators, and in relation to what is to be achieved by the year 2000.

Despite efforts in this second evaluation to provide the most realistic picture available of the global achievements based on national and regional evaluation reports, there were two constraints: (i) insufficient information concerning Member States' achievements in implementing their national strategies, which was supplemented, where possible, with information available within WHO and from other international sources; (ii) difficulties in comparing the achievements in 1990 with the earlier global monitoring and evaluation activities in 1983, 1985 and 1988, which led to revisions in the common framework and formats recommended for use by Member States and in the list of global indicators to be used for monitoring and evaluation of the strategy. A few additional indicators have also been included for the first time in the second evaluation with no baseline or earlier values for comparison.

In the first evaluation in 1985, one of the major problems identified by Member States in reporting their findings was the persistent deficiency of information support mechanisms for national health policy formulation and implementation, as well as for health systems development based on primary health care. In this second evaluation the reports contained more data on global HFA indicators, as well as additional findings concerning the implementation of the strategy. The statistical annex reflects this improvement in data availability and the present review has made use of those data that are relevant and of satisfactory quality, supplementing them with whatever data were available from other sources. Significant findings from the earlier chapters of this review are summarized below.

Progress and adequacy

Health systems development

Overall there has been strong political commitment to achieving health-for-all goals, and most countries have endorsed at the highest level the necessary policies and strategies (global indicator 1). Mechanisms to involve people are reported to be fully functioning or are being further developed in most countries (global indicator 2). Policy decisions have been taken in many countries, which has enabled them to mobilize at least central government resources for health (global indicator 3). However, in implementing the strategy the fundamental health-for-all policies and the principles applicable to health systems based on primary health care have not always been appropriately put into practice by the countries when attempting to facilitate universal access to essential health care with all eight essential elements of PHC on a continuing basis. The factors that slowed progress in implementing the strategy were: (i) the slow pace at which existing disease-control programmes have been reoriented towards people's needs; (ii) problems of collaboration to provide health care on a continuing basis through general health infrastructure; (iii) diffi-

culties in involving all those concerned (individuals, families, communities and local nongovernmental organizations as well as health personnel) in health care delivery; and (iv) weak management of health care delivery, especially at the operational level. The inadequate and uneven distribution of health personnel of different categories has frequently hindered the delivery of an appropriate mix of health care activities. The provision of effective health care directed to specific vulnerable groups and/or priority problems has not only been inhibited by lack of coordination and integration, but also possibly by lack of managerial expertise and creativity, including insufficient leadership from the ministry of health. Public health action may be confined to the national level and therefore limited in scope.

Health resources and their distribution

This section considers financial resources, human resources and health technology. The percentage of GNP spent on health is used as an indicator of the financial resources for health, including both public and private expenditure on health. Not many countries have provided information, and the available data are too limited to allow meaningful conclusions to be drawn. According to the available data there has been a slight increase in the percentage of GNP spent by central governments for health in all developing countries and most geographical regions. The per capita central government expenditure, however, shows a general fall in real spending in many developing countries. It should be noted that data on central government expenditure on health is difficult to compare among country groupings. There is also evidence that nongovernmental spending on health is becoming increasingly significant. Data on the percentage of national health expenditure devoted to local health services have been scarce (global indicator 4). However, for those countries for which data were available for both

Fig. 7.1
Framework for monitoring and evaluation of the strategy for health for all

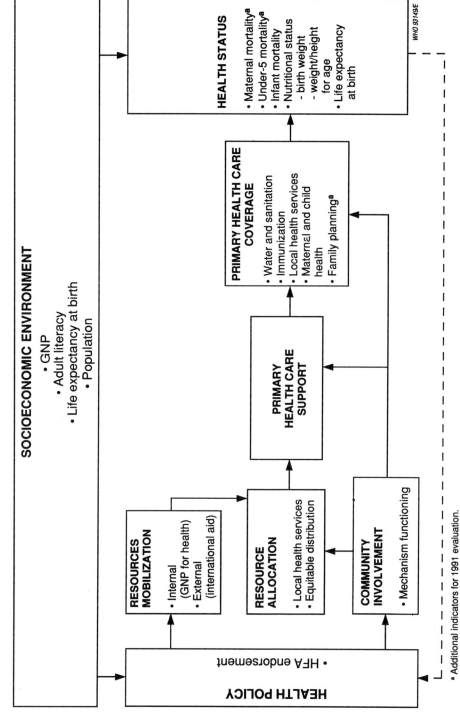

periods of time, the percentage has increased in developed countries, has been stagnant in the developing countries and has decreased in the least developed countries. Only a few countries have given information on global indicator 5 (equitable distribution of resources), and most of these are distributing resources more equitably. Even when countries report that the available resources are equitably distributed, there is little evidence that they are being used specifically to support services and activities at the peripheral level of the health system. Initiatives directed to priority problems and/or vulnerable groups have been launched, and specific programme activities to reduce inequities have been formulated. It is encouraging that many countries have started to review and reform the organization of their health care systems, including financing.

From the available data on human resources for health, it appears that, despite an excess of physicians in the developed and in some developing countries and a widespread shortage of nurses, the major problem continued to be the maldistribution of health personnel. There is increasing evidence that, as infrastructure expands, the means to use that infrastructure to provide care have been weak (e.g., not only is there a shortage of personnel, but in some cases even when appropriate personnel were available there was a logistic problem, such as lack of equipment, supplies, drugs, etc.). Many countries are reviewing the relevance of current medical education and assessing different factors which may influence professional behaviour (working situation and environment, status and remuneration). Many health programmes, however, continue to train health workers specifically to implement their programme activities and to achieve their particular programme targets.

Health technology used in primary health care is still inadequately assessed in most countries. Some countries reported the establishment of national research priorities related to major

diseases or to organizational issues such as human resources and finance. There is, however, no evidence to show that priority has been given to the choice of technology and methods appropriate for effective provision of essential care on a continuing basis through integration of preventive *and* promotive care with curative and rehabilitative services. This would have operational, financial and ethical implications as well as posing challenges for health professionals, training institutions and health managers.

Effectiveness and impact

This section assesses: (i) the effectiveness of action taken to develop health systems to increase coverage; and (ii) the impact of the strategy in terms of improvements in health status.

Health care coverage

Globally there have been significant increases in some of the subelements of primary health care (global indicator 7) since the first evaluation in 1985, such as immunization against the six target diseases of the Expanded Programme on Immunization, trained attendance at childbirth, local health services, and water supply and excreta-disposal facilities. Gaps between the developing and developed countries have been significantly reduced, although improvements in the least developed countries have been less satisfactory. Information on the percentage of the population covered by *all* elements of primary health care (global indicator 7) is not available. This indicator comprises four selected elements of primary health care, each of which may comprise several subelements (e.g., the fourth element of the indicator actually comprises two subelements: attendance by trained personnel for pregnancy and childbirth, *and* caring for children up to at least 1 year of age). Data may sometimes not even be available for *all* the subelements but only for one aspect of one subelement (e.g., trained personnel for childbirth). Similarly, data were available for safe water and excreta-disposal facilities separately, but not necessarily for both subelements. A review of the profile of coverages by the different subelements gives an unbalanced and distorted picture (Fig 7.2 and 7.3). For example, in the least developed countries around 1990, the coverage by trained personnel for antenatal care was 53%, yet immunization of pregnant women with tetanus toxoid vaccine was only 37%. Similarly the coverage for immunization varied from 43% to 79% for the various six target diseases, yet coverage for infant care was only 58%. These discrepancies indicate a lack of integration in the provision of essential health services.

Health status

During the last 10 years, significant improvements in health status as defined by such indicators as infant mortality rate (global indicator 9.1), life expectancy at birth (global indicator 10), and birthweight status (global indicator 8.1) have been noted. Infant mortality rates (IMR) decreased globally, more markedly in the developing countries than in the least developed countries. The gap in IMR that existed in 1980 between the developing and the developed countries has narrowed, while the gap between the least developed and the other developing countries has widened. Of the countries for which values for life expectancy at birth were available, the number of countries with a life expectancy over 60 years increased from 74 (total population, 2700 million) in 1980 to 91 (total population, 3600 million) in 1990. However, of the 37 least developed countries for which data were available for 1990, only one had an IMR below 50, and only two had a life expectancy at birth of over 60 years. Reductions in IMR and increases in life expectancy seem to be associated with the major gains made against vaccine-preventable diseases primarily targeted at infancy and early childhood. Nevertheless, there is increasing evidence that these improvements in life expectancy do not necessarily mean a healthier life. Moreover, increases in life expectancy have been consistently higher for females than for males. Also there has been virtually no improvement in the global situation as far as birthweight status is concerned.

For the second evaluation, two indicators were added: (i) maternal mortality rate (global indicator 9.2) and (ii) under-5 mortality rate (global indicator 9.3). Causes related to pregnancy and childbirth are among the leading causes of death for women of reproductive age; 99% of these deaths occur in developing countries. The under-5 mortality rate (the probability of a live born dying before the age of 5 years) was about six times higher for the developing countries than for developed market economies, and for the least developed countries about 11 times higher.

It is difficult to assess comprehensively health disparities between geographical areas, among different population groups and also in urban slums, since not enough data are available. There is, however, increasing evidence that such disparities have increased within countries since 1980.

Global socioeconomic environment

Education and income levels are associated with the development of health systems and health status. The indicators used to measure these levels have been the adult literacy rate (global indicator 11) and the per capita GNP (global indicator 12), which have increased globally, including in the developing countries, although not significantly for the least developed. The national socioeconomic environment, however, has not generally been conducive to the development of health systems based on primary health care, particularly where civil strife and sociopolitical instability have prevailed. Changes in priorities were also noted as a result

Fig. 7.2
Primary health care available at least for the essential elements, developing countries, 1983–1985 and 1988–1990

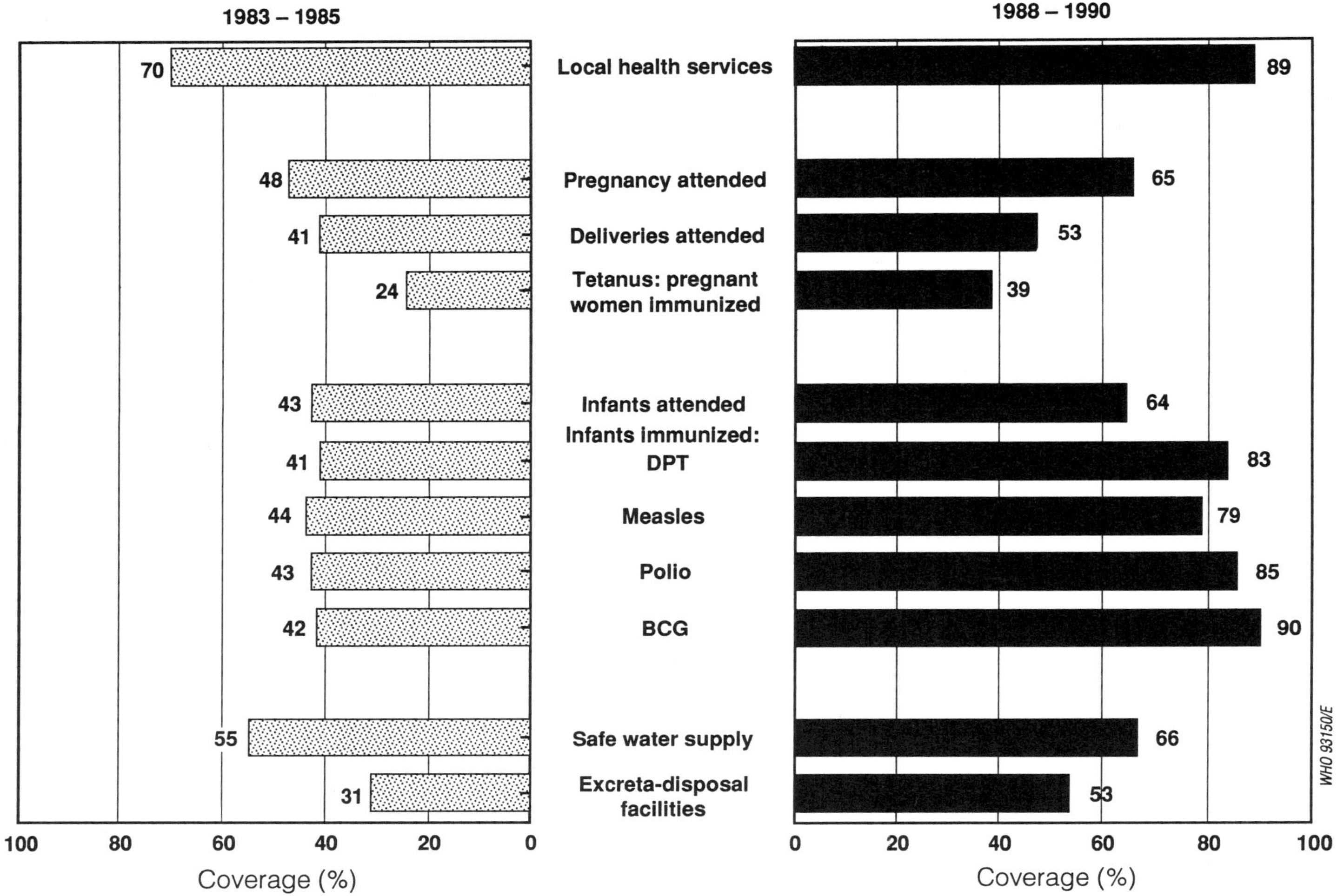

WHO 93150/E

1988 – 1990

Element	Coverage (%)
Local health services	89
Pregnancy attended	65
Deliveries attended	53
Tetanus: pregnant women immunized	39
Infants attended	64
Infants immunized: DPT	83
Measles	79
Polio	85
BCG	90
Safe water supply	66
Excreta-disposal facilities	53

Coverage (%)

1983 – 1985

Element	Coverage (%)
Local health services	70
Pregnancy attended	48
Deliveries attended	41
Tetanus: pregnant women immunized	24
Infants attended	43
Infants immunized: DPT	41
Measles	44
Polio	43
BCG	42
Safe water supply	55
Excreta-disposal facilities	31

Coverage (%)

143

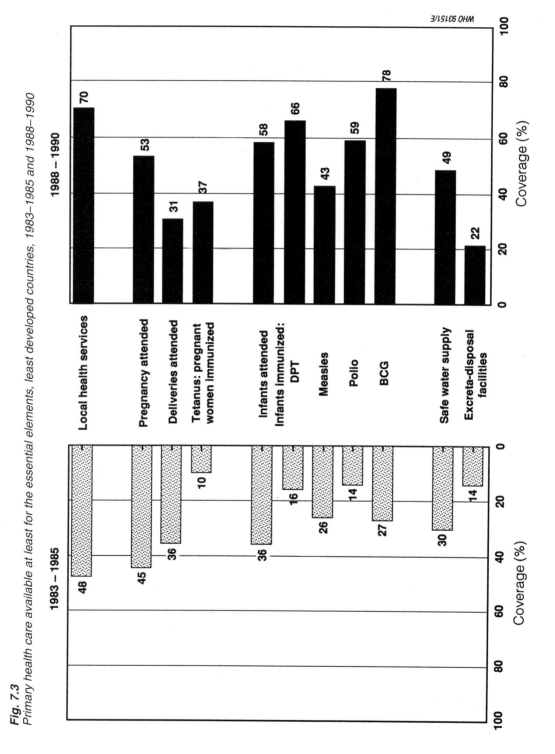

Fig. 7.3
Primary health care available at least for the essential elements, least developed countries, 1983–1985 and 1988–1990

WHO 93151/E

of the global recession, natural or manmade disasters and other emerging or new problems such as cholera and AIDS. The smooth implementation of national health-for-all strategies was sometimes hindered by certain groups representing specific interests at the expense of broader national priorities, including international technical and funding agencies.

There has been a noticeable trend among governments and international development agencies towards the recognition of people as the centre of development, and health as a basic component thereof. The social and political dimensions of development have also received more attention from international development organizations and agencies. The global environment is becoming more favourable to decision-making in health, given the general global trend towards democracy and freedom, initiatives such as universal literacy by the year 2000, and the integration of women in the mainstream of development policies. In health development there is a general trend towards more involvement of individuals, communities, professional groups and development agencies.

The global economic environment was unable to support sustainable national development owing to the slowing down of the pace of economic growth in the 1980s, increasing balance of payment problems in many countries, growing disparities in production performances in different parts of the world, and emerging new trade and foreign debt policies and practices.

Given the shrinking global availability of government resources, it has become increasingly evident that the developing countries, particularly the least developed countries, have been looking for ways of implementing policies and strategies that would enable them to make judicious use of the available national and international resources. There is also little evidence to show that the international funding agencies have shifted their aid predominantly towards low-income countries.

Overall assessment

The response by Member States to the second global evaluation of health-for-all strategies has been satisfactory, and data are now available on a larger number of global indicators than in 1985. Data and information on basic financial and human resources and on coverage by essential care with *all* eight essential elements of primary health care have not always been available; one of the factors which inhibited a more extensive analysis has been the lack of data on the global indicators in a disaggregated form for identifiable population groups.

Virtually every country is committed to health-for-all goals and endorsement at the highest level; national health policies and programmes have also been formulated in the framework of the Global Strategy. Mechanisms to facilitate community involvement in health are generally being developed, and in some countries resources are being more equitably distributed. Existing health services are being reoriented to a health system based on primary health care taking into account the role of the individual, family, community and local nongovernmental organizations, as well as health personnel.

During the period since the World Health Assembly adopted the Global Strategy and since the first evaluation, health status – as measured by such indicators as life expectancy and infant mortality – has improved globally. However, the pace of improvement has been slower for the least developed countries and, as a result, inequities between the developing and least developed countries are greater now than they were a decade ago.

The availability of essential health care has also increased globally. Yet, millions of people remain without access to either all or some elements of care. If the availability of certain elements of care increases, while the availability of other complementary elements does not, the positive impact on health status of the one can be offset by lack of the other. Similarly, if the infrastructure is expanded but the means to use that infrastructure to provide care is weak, no improvements in health status will be evident. In other words, in the development of health systems based on primary health care, the right things are being done, but not necessarily in all instances in the right form.

Worldwide, health systems development reflects increasingly the concepts, approaches and philosophy of primary health care. However, the health systems continue to give greater emphasis to specific diseases and conditions or to some elements of care and specific types of services (mostly vertical), which sometimes may not facilitate meeting the overall health needs of people at different phases of their lives on a continuing basis. Yet this ability of health systems to consider the needs of the individual as a person, i.e., the holistic view of health, is the very essence of health for all.

People are increasingly involved in improving their own health, which is one of the fundamental concepts of health for all, through specific health care measures taken by them as individuals and as members of families and communities, and by nongovernmental organizations and other health personnel. However, governments, the health sector and interest groups sometimes are reluctant to recognize the value of such contributions by individuals, nongovernmental organizations and health-related sectors and to establish real partnerships based on mutual respect and understanding.

In conclusion, it can be stated that improvements have been made in health status in terms of life expectancy at birth and infant mortality rates, and coverage levels by various elements of primary health care. Because such improvements seem to be more rapid in the developing countries than in the least developed ones, the disparities in health status between the developed and developing countries appear reduced but those between the least developed and other developing countries have increased. There is also some evidence that disparities in health status have increased within countries between certain population groups. Coverages by various elements of primary health care have been unbalanced and distorted in that although programmes have achieved their targets, their impact in terms of health status may not be significant. There is also little evidence that international and bilateral funding agencies have significantly shifted their aid priorities towards the low-income and/or least developed countries.

With the high-level commitment and endorsement of the Global Strategy and the establishment of mechanisms for involving people, a basis now exists for activities to implement the Strategy. However, it is not yet clear whether this has actually led to equitable distribution of resources and to shifting the available resources to support local health services. There is, however, evidence that the health sector has been able to mobilize at least central government resources, in spite of unfavourable economic constraints domestically and internationally. A major problem has been ineffective cooperation between programmes within the health sector and insufficient coordination with other sectors. Many countries have been developing innovative ways of financing health care, reviewing their medical education and training programmes for health personnel, and revising disease control programmes so that they have a more holistic, interdisciplinary and intersectoral, approach ensuring global collaboration in support of health protection and provision.

Reference

1. World Health Assembly resolution WHA34.36; and *Global strategy for health for all by the year 2000*. Geneva, World Health Organization, 1981 ("Health for All" Series, No. 3).

CHAPTER 8

Outlook for the future

Introduction

The purpose of this concluding chapter is to draw from the preceding chapters the major lessons from this evaluation, particularly the accumulated evidence of progress and problems as reported from the countries. This information will then be used to identify likely future trends (generally to the year 2000), the major issues which these trends imply, and the resulting challenges to be addressed in the continuing effort to achieve national and global health-for-all goals and targets. These issues and challenges call for a new agenda of national and international action in health.

In identifying likely future trends in health, two kinds of environments have been considered, the "external environment" which provides to the health sector a variety of opportunities for and threats to national health-for-all strategy development and implementation, and the "internal environment" characterized by the strengths and weaknesses within the health sector currently reported by countries in this evaluation.

Quantitative projections have been made for only a few of these variables. Most of the trends result from less sophisticated analysis amounting to a global review and accumulation of various types of health system accomplishments and difficulties within the changing political and economic environments of today. The major source of the information has been the country and regional evaluation reports and summaries of them appearing in earlier chapters. However,

this has been supplemented by a review of recent health and development literature in order to strengthen the health trends and projections.

The estimates of what is likely to happen within the next decade are only educated guesses at best, very often no more than the extension of current trends with some hypotheses as to the causes of these trends and how the causal factors may change in the future. The subjective judgements of likely future tendencies in health policy, organization, and management are derived from prevailing national and international opinion, mixed with a sprinkling of logic, and hope.

The purpose of this guess at the future is to highlight those factors which deserve attention, either because they represent positive change (opportunities and strengths) which should be pursued and maximized in the years to come, or because they are conditions (threats and weaknesses) which will become considerably worse if no action is taken.

The report of the second monitoring of health-for-all progress had identified five critical challenges in 1988. This evaluation provides an update of those challenges, and identifies specific tasks to be undertaken by governments and by the international community, including WHO. These tasks are felt to be important as the collective membership of WHO accelerates the implementation of the Strategy for health for all.

Emphasis will be placed on the fact that people are central to health development. The process of human development, the well-being of the individual and the importance of people's involvement in, and their assuming responsibility for, the maintenance of their own health all comprise a central theme of this concluding chapter. There is a need to empower people with information, ideas and responsibility, and to encourage free expression of concern and individual and community action to solve health-related problems.

Assessment of future trends

Economic growth is at a rather low level in most of the world, with a fluctuating world economy, and current health-financing systems can no longer cope with the demands made on them, even in affluent countries. There are signs that a substantial improvement in real net resource flows towards Africa and the LDCs is unlikely. These trends are sure to have negative consequences for human development, including health, in many countries.

These future trends will now be examined under six headings: socioeconomic development, health status, development of health systems, health care, health resources, and health and the environment.

Future trends in socioeconomic development

Growth in the world economy decreased from more than 4% in 1985 to 3% in 1990, and economic growth of the developed countries is expected to continue at this lower level. Growth prospects for the developing countries vary from optimistic to disastrous, being fastest in the rapidly industrializing countries of east Asia, but growth is expected to continue to be slow in sub-Saharan Africa, parts of Latin America and the Caribbean and other countries of Asia. On balance, resources are currently flowing from the developing to the developed countries, a condition which is expected to continue.

A World Bank forecast predicts that the incidence of poverty in the developing world as a whole will fall, but the number of poverty-stricken people in sub-Saharan Africa will rise by 85 million to reach 265 million by the end of the century.

The average annual population growth rate, running at 1.73% per year in 1990–1995, will decline slowly to 0.99% in 2020–2025. But in spite of a falling birth rate in the group of developing countries as a whole, world population is projected to increase by almost one-fifth, from 5300 million to 6300 million, during the next decade. Almost all of this growth will occur in developing countries, where annual growth rates are expected to average about 2.1%. This will be accompanied by continued rapid urbanization in those countries. The urban population is expected to rise from 45% of the total global population in 1990 to 51% by the year 2000. Eighteen cities in the Third World will have populations greater than 10 million. Total population growth rates as well as urban growth rates will be highest in Africa. This growth of population often erases the gains made in health service coverage; although the percentage of coverage increases, the absolute numbers of people without coverage continue to rise.

Globally, the proportion of the population aged 65 and over is projected to increase from 6.2% in 1990 to 6.8% in the year 2000, which implies that there will be an additional 96 million elderly citizens to care for, 70 million of whom will be in developing countries.

The Office of the United Nations High Commissioner for Refugees (UNHCR) estimates that as at January 1991 there were more than 17 million refugees globally. It is reported by UNHCR that 28 million refugees have been assisted by various international agencies over the past 40 years. The relaxation of restraints on movement by many governments (in eastern Europe, for example) could for a time result in an expanding flow of refugees which will generate pressures for services, including health services.

There is an immense potential for positive effects of education on the health of populations. The increase in primary school enrolment will lead to dramatic rises in literacy rates in the developing world, which will translate into improved family hygiene. Despite this, from the expected population growth it may be surmised that the number of illiterate people in the world, which was around 950 million in 1985, may well reach 1000 million by the end of the century.

According to the United Nations, the female literacy rate in developing countries was still only 50% in 1985, compared to 71% for men. Enrolment rates for girls have been increasing rapidly and in 1989 had reached 90% of the rate for boys. It is expected that during the coming decade there will be further enhancement of women's status, equipping them with basic knowledge and skills, giving them access to services, and bringing them into the mainstream of development as more equal partners. That being said, UNESCO reports that there are about 500 million illiterate women in rural areas who have little chance of improving their education.

The tendency towards more democratic forms of government will lead to increasing calls by the people for more equitably distributed, better-quality services, for a stronger voice in decisions on priorities and for the means of obtaining health services. The spread of education in combination with the trend towards more democracy and participation in decision-making will intensify demands for more objective and understandable information about health, health technology and necessary health services, and pressure to complement the role of the health professions in health care decision-making.

Computing power and telecommunications will continue to expand around the world, bringing more information rapidly to more people. This will help to improve health in two ways: (i) by facilitating research and health service delivery; (ii) by bringing more preventive, promotive and curative information to the general public. This expansion of public information on health and health technology, however, may raise public expectations of improved health care excessively, far exceeding what can possibly be made available to all in the near future.

The conflict between macroeconomic, industrial, energy and agricultural policies and the need to protect the public from the unhealthy side-effects of some of these policies will continue, but there is growing evidence that the people's voice is being heard and that their health concerns are increasingly being taken into account by development planners.

Future trends in health status

The United Nations Population Division projects that life expectancy at birth for the world as a whole will rise to about 68 years in the year 2000. The projected increase for developing countries is likely to be twice that of the developed world because they started at a lower level. The gains in developing countries primarily reflect the expected decline in infant mortality rates to 60 per 1000 by the year 2000. However, improvements in infant and child mortality are expected to be more modest in sub-Saharan Africa than in east Asia and Latin America, largely because of the AIDS pandemic.

The projected decline in infant (including perinatal) and child mortality is to a large extent based on the assumptions of sustained, if slow, improvement in socioeconomic conditions and future expansion of coverage with effective health technologies such as family planning, immunization, oral rehydration, and appropriate treatment for acute respiratory infection. The success of these interventions in recent years suggests that there are some grounds for further optimism in countries where coverage is low but is expected to increase.

The following brief survey of health trends focuses on the most significant causes of mortality and morbidity, particularly in the developing world.

The leading causes of illness and death in many developing countries are the **respiratory diseases**. As childhood deaths from the vaccine-preventable diseases have been falling, the proportion of total deaths caused by acute respiratory infections, including pneumonia, has been increasing. However, a simple method has been developed by which a mother or local health worker can recognize when a child with such an infection needs treatment, and standardized antibiotic regimens have been established. If these can be implemented in as widespread a fashion as immunization and oral rehydration, the prospects are good that the consequences of acute respiratory infections can eventually be reduced.

Diarrhoeal diseases are another major cause of ill health and death in the developing world. Although there are treatments for these diseases, little progress can be made as long as the patients return to their insanitary environment to be infected again. The final report of the International Drinking Water Supply and Sanitation Decade (1980–1990) showed that even if financial resources could be assured at the same level as the extraordinarily high one achieved during the Decade, population growth will exceed the expansion of those services.

The **malaria** situation is stationary in many areas and deteriorating in others, particularly in new settlements. Strengthening malaria control programmes that have been allowed to deteriorate will not be enough, given the spreading drug resistance of the parasite and insecticide resistance of the vector. Effective vaccines are still a long way off. China has, however, achieved notable success in reducing malaria mortality by basing a widespread network of malaria clinics on a good health infrastructure, and continually evaluating the efficacy of drug regimens.

Regarding **malnutrition**, only long-term changes in food security, backed by good nutri-

tion education programmes, will make a permanent difference. Emergency food aid is soon gone, but damage to the protein-deprived growing brain is permanent, as is stunting. However, village studies in Nepal have shown that even illiterate mothers can learn to feed their children local foods that reduce the incidence of vitamin A deficiency and associated blindness. If this type of initiative becomes widespread in the next decade, the malnutrition situation will improve. Obesity shows an upward trend, but in many developed countries people are beginning to watch their diets and protect themselves from overweight and the accompanying disorders of hypertension, heart disease, diabetes, gastrointestinal problems and various bone and joint diseases.

The number of cases of **pulmonary tuberculosis** will continue to rise because of reactivation of the disease in individuals infected with human immunodeficiency virus (HIV). A large proportion of these patients may in turn spread tuberculosis further. New drug regimens are available, but the ideal, single-dose medication has not yet been developed. However, the prospects for tuberculosis control have vastly improved with the increased cure rates achieved through new patient-management strategies and short-course chemotherapy (6 months).

Chronic **obstructive lung disease**, which includes chronic bronchitis and emphysema, is a major killer. Its causes are cigarette smoking, air pollution, biomass and high-sulfur fuels, and vehicle-exhaust emissions. The situation will get worse before it gets better, since although air pollution controls and antismoking legislation are being implemented in the developed countries, unregulated tobacco smoking and polluting industries are increasing in developing countries as they in turn industrialize without such controls and their population explosion leads to even more smoking, and to cooking and home heating with biomass and other cheap, polluting fuels.

Nearly 90% of the projected **HIV infections**

and acquired immunodeficiency syndrome (AIDS) cases for this decade will be in the developing countries. In sub-Saharan Africa alone, WHO projects that some 10 million HIV-infected infants will be born by the year 2000, and 10 million children will be orphaned by the death of their parents from AIDS. During this decade and the next, the projected deaths from AIDS may increase child mortality rates in some countries by as much as 50%, wiping out the gains made in child survival over the past two decades. In Asia the pandemic is still at an early stage, but indications are that it is growing quickly. The transmission of infection will increasingly take place through heterosexual intercourse, which will be the source of 75–80% of all cases in the year 2000, rather than through homosexual intercourse and drug abuse.

Among adults, **cardiovascular diseases** will remain the leading cause of death during the next decade, in line with the progressive aging of the population and the adoption of unhealthy lifestyles. But although the total number of deaths from cardiovascular diseases will remain high worldwide, in most developed countries there has been a decline in the rates for these diseases, and this will continue as people improve their lifestyles.

Despite the expected progress in the early detection and treatment of **cancer**, it will be an increasingly important cause of death among adults, in developing as well as developed countries. This increase will be associated with the aging population, environmental pollution, and the spread of unhealthy lifestyles. Perhaps the most significant of the last-named is tobacco use, which is a major risk factor for the principal chronic diseases including chronic obstructive lung disease (see above) as well as lung cancer. If current trends continue, global tobacco-related mortality will increase from about 3 million now to 10 million in the 2020s, with the vast majority of these deaths occurring in developing countries. As smoking becomes as common among women as it has been among men,

lung cancer is overtaking breast cancer as the leading cause of cancer for women in some countries.

There are prospects that **mental illness** will continue to increase in view of the stresses caused by the disruption of old ways of life, as agricultural countries industrialize and rural people continue to crowd into the cities. Institutions for the mentally ill consume a large proportion of the public health budget in some countries, and ways to reduce this burden, for instance by moving some patients into care by the local community, will be explored by many countries.

Mortality and disabilities due to **traffic accidents** will rise further in many developing countries when the growth in the number of motor vehicles outstrips the provision of new roadworks and safety measures. As industrialization proceeds in the developing world without adequate safeguards for workers' health, **accidents at work** will increase, and so will major **technological disasters** such as those which have already occurred in the nuclear, chemical and oil industries (tanker spills) and which are likely to affect large populations and the environment.

There is some progress, however. The childhood **immunization** strategy is working. Endemic transmission of wild poliovirus may have already stopped in the hemisphere of the Americas, and prospects for the global eradication of poliomyelitis by the year 2000 remain good *provided that the increased funding needs can be met.* Immunization rates are expected to increase during the decade, leading to further reductions in illness and death due to vaccine-preventable diseases, prominent among them being measles, neonatal tetanus and whooping cough. The World Summit for Children has given a boost to child immunization (as well as to a broad range of other health interventions). The programme components and management are tried and tested, and the resources required to sustain the immunization initiative are likely to be available thanks to massive support by international agencies, nongovernmental organizations and governments.

There are other **vaccines** available, some of which are being added to the childhood immunization schedule in countries where they are appropriate. They include vaccines against yellow fever, hepatitis B and Japanese encephalitis in some developing countries, and vaccines against mumps, rubella and haemophilus influenza B in developed countries. For epidemiological reasons they will not lead to the eradication of all these diseases; however, they will markedly decrease illness and death caused by them. A major international effort to accelerate the development of new vaccines and to facilitate the application of the existing ones has been launched by WHO, UNICEF, UNDP, the World Bank and the Rockefeller Foundation under the title of the Children's Vaccine Initiative. This initiative will further contribute to the role immunization can play in reducing morbidity and mortality.

New **drugs** from pharmaceutical research and biotechnology are coming on to the market, and new uses for old ones are being found. For example, ivermectin is providing an invaluable complement to vector control efforts in preventing blindness in the West African Onchocerciasis Programme, and is now being introduced alone in other endemic areas where vector control is not being applied. Multidrug therapy has led to the first recorded reduction in the number of registered leprosy patients. The faster these new products and applications can be brought into widespread use, the sooner an improvement in the health situation will be seen – but widespread use in developing countries will basically depend on price, as well as on an efficient delivery system.

The application of simple **technology** to provide clean water has resulted in a dramatic decline in the incidence of guinea-worm infection in India and Pakistan, where it is expected to be eliminated shortly, and similar progress in West Africa has led to the target date of 1995 being set for global guinea-worm eradication.

Future trends in the development of health systems

There has been a widespread trend towards decentralization in health management from the central level to regions, provinces and districts. This is a policy and organizational change which, when undertaken, usually extends across most government sectors. Therefore it is likely to continue. However, the true extent of devolution of authority, responsibility and resources is not always clear, nor is the effectiveness of such decentralization.

Throughout the country-evaluation reports runs a continuous thread regarding the burning need to strengthen management skills in order to proceed with implementation. And indeed, during the reporting period the number and types of health management training activities grew considerably. Gradually it is being recognized that management strengthening requires more than training, and that health management must be closely integrated with the programme subject being managed. It is projected that the desire for improving performance and quality will lead to other styles of management strengthening, including procedures review and revision, and in-service problem-solving.

Two trends deserve specific mention. The move to enhance community involvement has been widespread. There is some question as to how effective and sustainable are the various types of community involvement and how much more can be expected from communities, particularly those in the least developed countries.

The second trend relates to integration. It has been more difficult to obtain consensus on this health service concept than on any other. Most health programmes which have received special funding and management have achieved varying degrees of success, but they have been accused of verticalization and are being encouraged to integrate their activities and support. While this is occurring, the strengths of these programmes should not be lost, and in fact such programmes offer a point of entry for strengthening the management of primary health care while increasing practical integration of services. Further integration of services will occur, particularly at the peripheral level, but each country will be devising an approach which is most appropriate in its circumstances for ensuring that all its people receive basic minimum care with sufficient quality to make it effective.

Health status is the outcome of many different developmental and behavioural activities. It is therefore the shared responsibility of development sectors, rather than the responsibility of the health sector alone, and depends upon effective coordination between them. Clear understanding by other related sectors of the concept and practice of health development is very important in enhancing health development as part of socioeconomic development. Unfortunately, in many countries this understanding is still weak, and the situation may not be easy to solve in the short term. In addition, the health sector will increasingly need to support the goals of other sectors in order to help achieve balanced development.

There are few examples of countries in which extensive and continuing intersectoral coordination for health is taking place. Many specialized organizational mechanisms for improving coordination have been established, but many soon became defunct or operate with little benefit, particularly intersectoral councils and committees at the central level. There may well be a need to return to the simplified coordination mechanisms more traditionally used for communications between government agencies. It has been observed that the participation of the private sector and nongovernmental organizations in planned health development is growing, and their participation is expected to dramatically expand in the 1990s. There may also be a revival of special intersectoral development projects and programmes which combine the efforts of several sectors in addressing a multipurpose development objective, benefiting a particular geographical area or target group. While such approaches have diminished in popularity in recent years, their implementation success and modest cost per beneficiary should lead to their being reconsidered for certain purposes.

Many countries commented on the problems of managing international cooperation in health. While the total amount of cooperation is likely to continue to grow, there is the implication that the inadequate coordination and varying technical quality of external collaboration in health requires urgent attention by all governments and agencies. Ministries will demand and obtain a louder voice in the programming and management of external support. Agencies will have to propose more innovative styles of collaboration which bring effective technologies and learning processes under the control of national administrations and institutions, thereby increasing sustainability. A related issue is the number of least developed countries whose developmental and operational resources for health come predominantly from external sources, which creates a continuing situation of dependency.

Future trends in health care

The quantitative indicators of coverage with the essential elements of primary health care have for the most part demonstrated steady increases since the first evaluation. These range from coverage with safe water and excreta-disposal facilities to antenatal and infant care and immunization. The availability of local health services has risen to almost 90% of the population in developing countries, attesting to the success in efforts to expand health infrastructure. Although the trend is significant, the validity of the coverage figures is sometimes questionable as there is little information on the equity of accessibility to the services and on their quality.

There may be a slowing of the improvement in coverage for two reasons. Firstly, the funds from both national and international sources for infrastructure expansion may decline. Secondly, it is always harder to reach the last 10–20% of the population, even though these are usually the groups that most need the health care. Nevertheless, the original primary health care coverage goals are within reach, if the political and programme commitment is maintained and more resources are directed towards vulnerable groups.

The trend in expansion of curative services will continue to be strong, but this need not be at the expense of preventive and promotive services, if such services can increasingly be provided from curative care settings. On the other hand, the expanding private sector may take some of the load off the public curative services. This may allow governments to concentrate their resources and attention more on prevention and promotion.

Future trends in health resources

Human resources

The deficiency most often cited by countries was shortage of qualified health manpower. This is despite the fact that manpower of all types has been growing faster than operating budgets. The problem of the inappropriate mix and distribution of health manpower is also growing. The current imbalances between physicians and nurses and other paramedical and technological staff will become more and more widespread. The government health services in many countries suffer from low productivity due to poor working conditions, low pay and lack of career opportunities, which lead to low motivation, reduced performance, and a high wastage rate. It is unlikely that there can be rapid increases in government health manpower or salaries owing to the limited growth possibilities of operating budgets, so these problems will continue. More countries will prepare manpower plans in the hope that the economic situation will improve, or in order to cope with restricted budgets. Problems with inappropriate curricula in training institutions will take many years to correct, and vested interests will continue to oppose the changes. Professional freedom will increasingly be monitored and questioned by those who pay for the services. However, some countries, particularly in Asia, are concentrating on training paramedical staff rather than more physicians, as well as upgrading existing staff and providing incentives for work in rural areas. These measures should lead to an improvement in coverage and quality of care.

Financial resources

Structural adjustment policies in many developing countries may continue to imply tight government control over expenditures on health and social services, often to the detriment of poorer populations who depend upon government services. However, the effect of structural adjustment has not been the same in all developing countries. While some countries have had to cut back, this has often occurred in capital development budgets, which reduces the cuts to operating funds. Some developing countries have not reduced government health expenditure at all.

During the evaluation period there was a dramatic increase of national interest in experimenting with and developing various health financing schemes. Health insurance, social security and various fee-for-service and community-support mechanisms were mentioned. This trend will continue. The evaluation has disclosed that resources have often not been redirected towards new health priorities and those most in need. This suggests that many governments will need to develop new strategies and programmes which focus attention and resources on special target groups (rural and urban poor, minority groups).

The health sector will have to make prudent use of the available resources by cutting down misplaced allocations, sharpening priorities, and implementing policies and strategies that improve effectiveness and impact and reduce waste. Cost-consciousness will become an issue of increasing importance within the health sectors of developing countries as it has in the developed countries. Health authorities will have to stress "healthy policies", for example: discouraging smoking through raised prices and education and agricultural policies instead of reliance on treatment of the effects of smoking; and promotion of safer highways through healthy road policies instead of building more facilities for the injured.

Harder to solve will be the concentration of government health resources in major curative institutions. The requirement for maintaining the levels of operating funds for these institutions limits the amount of reallocation that is possible. Growth in the different areas of nongovernmental health services (modern and traditional) as well as not-for-profit health sources of finance or service provision (such as religious or charitable concerns), may take some pressure off the government. The government will retain primary responsibility for ensuring that the needs of the underprivileged are met, and for coordinating different elements of the public/private mix towards overall health policy objectives. New and less directive mechanisms will be sought to promote a greater harmony of interests among different health care institutions.

Science and technology

Research in vaccines, pharmaceuticals and medical equipment is becoming ever more expensive, with the result that the end-products are priced out of the reach of developing countries. Yet pressures from manufacturers and donors to adopt these costly new technologies, and even from the general public, are intense. The trend seems to be towards more and more expensive treatments for diseases affecting fewer and fewer people. However, the problem of costly essential vaccines will be addressed by mobilizing private and public sector support to develop new and improved vaccines for children under the auspices of the Children's Vaccine Initiative.

The new gene technologies will first be targeted towards the treatment of diseases for which there are markets in developed countries. Because there is no rich market in developing countries, the big multinational drug and medical supply and equipment companies, with notable exceptions, have shown little interest in developing the low-cost products for which those countries are crying out.

Yet basic, appropriate technology does exist. Oral rehydration salts are cheap and effective. Bednets impregnated with the insecticide permethrin protect against malaria. The WHO basic radiology system is economical, robust, easy to maintain and practical. In general, it is hoped that research and development will generate new and improved preventive, therapeutic and enabling technologies, giving attention to simplicity and adaptability, to meet the needs of developing countries.

Future trends in health and the environment

It can be predicted that because of past and ongoing deterioration of the environment, including deforestation and misuse of land, floods and drought are likely to be more frequent in the coming decade. The people in developing countries inevitably are less prepared for these situations and are less able to respond to them. It is expected that more attention will be given to disaster preparedness planning, pre-positioning of disaster supplies and other preparatory measures which will reduce the damage to property and health caused by disasters.

Water resources for human, agricultural and industrial use are diminishing around the world. Yet the world's growing population demands ever more water. Pollution of land with toxic wastes is followed by their seepage into the water supply. Pollution of water with human wastes is followed by the spread of disease. Pollution of the air with sulfur and nitrous oxides and other pollutants leads to respiratory problems. The hesitant measures now being taken to limit emissions and control these problems will take much longer than the next decade to have a noticeable effect, but at least they will go some way towards protecting the health of future generations.

Strategic issues

It is clear from the previous chapters that progress towards health for all is being made on many fronts. Probably the greatest single achievement of health for all so far is the almost universal policy endorsement given to this aim. The WHO Constitution, the resolutions of the World Health Assembly, and various international proclamations supporting primary health care all confirm health as a fundamental human right and have indicated that health for all is in reality a search for social justice and equity. It is clear that these global pronouncements have gradually been integrated within most national health policies and legislation around the world. This policy endorsement is reconfirmed by the present evaluation and can be expected to modify the trends in the health and health-related sectors compared with those recently observed. This gives cause for optimism about the chances of achieving the goal.

Even so, the evaluation and trend assessment discloses a number of issues which demand increasing attention in the future if sustained progress towards health for all is to be maintained. There has been general recognition by Member States of the need to further accelerate the implementation of their health-for-all strategies. The investment made thus far, both nationally and internationally, is considerable. The performance and effect of these investments must be improved.

It is evident that every national health system should have certain basic components.

Firstly, health for all means there should be an equitable distribution of resources, equal access to services and increased equity in health. Secondly, the system must recognize the right of each individual to quality health care throughout life. Thirdly, the system must generate and distribute the resources needed to prevent or take care of the health problems in each phase of the life cycle. The responsibility of individuals and their community in determining their own health and welfare is a theme which must receive even more emphasis in the future.

The following paragraphs discuss five categories of issues confronting future health development. These issues are chosen to summarize the results of this second evaluation in a manner that focuses attention on the *acceleration of implementation*, i.e., getting on with the job that remains to be done to achieve the object of health for all, bearing in mind that people are central to health development.

Clarifying the roles of governments and communities

It has long been recognized that health must be considered within the wider context of overall socioeconomic development; there is now growing realization that human development must be at the core of all social and economic development processes. How do these two major challenges affect the manner in which governments and communities must define their future responsibility in health development?

What are the most appropriate government roles in health?

In the face of limited public resources for health development and maintenance, and limited capacity to administer, many governments will find it necessary to undertake a serious redefinition of their responsibility within the health sector. It is probable that the direct administration of medical services by central government will give way to more decentralized and pluralistic modes of regulation, and of finance. The expansion of private practice and hospitals which is taking place in countries at all levels of development should be recognized and regulated. Altering responsibility in this fashion may offer the opportunity to strengthen the government-supported public health prevention and promotion functions, which are of little interest to the private sector. Many governments must strive to develop equitable health financing schemes and ensure there are special care programmes for those with the least physical access and financial means.

The monitoring and control of the quality of both public and private health care is a task of growing importance. Intensive review and revision of health legislation and regulations are needed. Many countries will introduce social legislation to ensure the health rights of the underprivileged. All governments will be seeking ways to increase effective interaction between health and other sectors in order to make health promotion and protection a concern of all public and private endeavours. In addition, government health administrations will increasingly be called upon to support human development through programmes in other sectors and thus not focus only on health and social services.

How to enable individuals and communities to determine their most appropriate role in self-care and community health development

The health rights and responsibilities of the individual must receive growing attention. Increased efforts are needed to enable citizens to take more responsibility for maintaining their own health, principally by providing them with effective information on health protection and self-care. The health professions must improve the way in which they inform the public about risks, interventions, the scope for self-care and the potential for community action. The means for effective community health action and control which can be built into community func-

tions in a sustainable manner are still to be found. Health care and development must increasingly come under community patronage; governments must devise ways to facilitate such community health management. There must be more international effort to produce health information for the public.

All of this suggests that many governments should develop and promote new styles of community involvement which incorporate realism and information into their promotion of and support for community health action. Indeed, fostering healthy communities should be considered an investment in socioeconomic development with a high potential for return.

How to strengthen the mananagement of health development and health technology

How to strengthen health leadership and management capability

New approaches are needed for strengthening the management of public health and health care, which recognize that management practice and skills cannot be developed as a separate discipline, but must be integrated within the health care administration and practice of a country. This implies that the process of management strengthening will depend less upon traditional training approaches, but will rather be accomplished more often by means of learning through action in problem situations, and by means of review and revision of service procedures.

Health leadership will be less concerned with promotion and advocacy of health-for-all strategies, and will rather address the impediments to strategy and programme implementation. Many existing sectoral and intersectoral guidance and coordination mechanisms are not effective and must be revitalized and consolidated for the sake of efficiency and effective programme implementation.

Intersectoral approaches to health development are needed which combine effective strategies from several sectors into manageable intersectoral development programmes. Often these intersectoral activities will be implemented at subnational levels or be directed towards specific population groups.

Finally, health management must be seen as both a technical and administrative enterprise which requires better information in a number of areas: technological, epidemiological, community perspectives, professional attitudes, environmental trends, financial and personnel status, and indicators of service performance, quality and efficiency.

How to strengthen health technology development and health information and focus them on national health priorities

Appropriate technology is needed at district and peripheral levels and in the communities to help close the equity gap. While health research and development capabilities are expected to increase, especially in developing countries, health research resources are inadequately focused on the priority needs for appropriate health technology, and on developing effective strategies for the implementation of primary health care. New research priorities must be aimed at equity, lifestyle, quality of care and the environment, as well as priority health problems such as AIDS, malaria and cardiovascular disease.

The effectiveness of certain standard technologies commonly provided within primary health care must be confirmed and continually monitored. Evaluation of the implementation and effectiveness of primary health care and their improvement could benefit from more candour, particularly when assessing the more common approaches such as decentralization, integration, community participation and the use of community health workers.

There is a growing appreciation of the need to develop a better understanding of the health of underprivileged populations. More and better information is needed to define the size, location and conditions of the least privileged in order that programmes can be directed towards rectifying current inequities in the health of the population. Health research and evaluation must be refocused to address these information needs.

It is generally admitted that both technical and public health information are inadequate in most countries. Strengthening epidemiological surveillance and analysis is an urgent priority, as is facilitating the appropriate use of existing case and community data maintained by health services. Improved indicators for monitoring health and managing health services must be developed and incorporated in the information systems.

Reorientation of health care systems to focus on priority needs

How to focus health systems on priority population groups and their health problems

While international and national health policy promotion and development have achieved a certain degree of success in mobilizing interest and action for achieving universal coverage with primary health care, reorientation must now focus squarely on ensuring that care is available to those priority population groups currently most in need and with least access. Attention must also be focused upon major and growing health problems and risk factors, particularly those affecting the least advantaged population groups. The health problems to be given priority should include those diseases close to eradication, those which can be solved with effective preventive and control technologies, and those expected to worsen in the coming years because of changing demographic, social, economic, and epidemiological conditions. AIDS, malaria, tuberculosis, cardiovascular diseases, substance abuse, nutrition and pollution will be among such priority concerns. The necessary focus on priority problems and population groups must be achieved, while avoiding the separate delivery of service activities, as sometimes occurs when certain health activities benefit from special funding and management.

The reorientation of the health system must include a redefinition of the responsibilities of the government and private health sectors mentioned above, with attention on how best to promote health, prevent disease and efficiently manage expensive curative care processes.

Quality assurance in preventive and curative services will take on added importance as higher levels of coverage are achieved. The need for improvement in quality is greatest at the peripheral service levels, such as health centres and district hospitals. Quality improvement must be addressed by strengthening procedures to ensure that essential tasks are performed correctly.

How to improve the production and use of human resources for health

Several predominant themes must receive attention in future efforts to develop human resources for health. Improving training processes, methods and materials will be a continuing theme, particularly as priority primary health care tasks will be given more emphasis by all categories of staff. Raising the sense of public responsibility in all aspects of health care, with quality improvement as the ultimate objective, must be another central theme. Staff for the support of priority areas and population groups should be more carefully allocated, since increasing the numbers of health personnel may not always be possible. Manpower use must be rationalized to ensure better correlation between the type of service to be provided and the type of staff to be assigned. In addition, attention must be given to ensuring that the technical and material support required by health professionals is available (supplies, equipment, logistics, communications). All efforts to strengthen health manpower must emphasize the need for "humanizing" health care.

It is likely that the expansion of private sources of health care and the greater involvement of nongovernmental organizations will complicate the process of health personnel administration, including the registration of all qualified staff. Nevertheless, systems for health personnel administration must be improved in order for governments to adequately oversee the production and use of this valuable resource. Finally, improved career development schemes are needed in order to increase the productivity of health personnel while addressing the disparity that often exists between the salaries of health staff in the public and private sectors.

Health financing

How to design and implement appropriate health financing mechanisms with special concern for populations in greatest need

It is proving difficult to develop efficient health care financing schemes in countries with wide disparities in public earning capacity. There needs to be a more active international exchange of ideas and of experience in innovative health financing schemes. While inequity is a problem to be dealt with in this context, increasing attention must be given to finding the optimum effective funding level for health care that is responsive both to real health needs and to the requirements of efficiency. Cost control will become an increasing concern in developing countries in both the public and private sectors.

Resource mobilization will remain a major preoccupation in the health sector, with health financing schemes, including fee-for-service and health insurance, being only partial solutions at best. In any case, health care financing in any country will normally require a combination of schemes. The redefinition of government responsibility in health may allow some shifting of resources from costly curative care towards health prevention and promotion.

International cooperation

How to increase the amount and effectiveness of international cooperation for health development, while giving priority to the least developed countries

The frequent mention in country reports of the deficiencies in international collaboration in health should challenge countries and international agencies alike to develop improved types of collaboration. It will be important that receiving governments strengthen their coordination of external support while being aware of the best that each external agency has to offer. Sustainability must be the watchword in collaboration.

In particular, WHO will be faced with the challenge posed by these implementation issues. WHO must nurture its promotion of health for all with realism and practical support. New styles of collaboration must be devised that ensure that all support is of a high technical quality, and is adjusted to the evolving country situations and constraints. The formulation of WHO support to countries must be given more thoughtful attention jointly by governments and the Organization. WHO country offices must be strengthened technically and managerially. Basic public health practice must be re-emphasized in WHO's collaborative programmes, along with health care financing and the strengthening of important health care support systems. There is also a growing need to improve coordination in health action across the United Nations system and among all agencies concerned.

As WHO succeeds in strengthening its technical cooperation at country level it will simultaneously strengthen its other role as the directing and coordinating authority in international health work. Emphasis must be given to the coordination of research, to the broad dissemination of information on new technology and development approaches, to setting of standards, and to maintainance of specialized expertise in priority health development subjects.

Finally, it is important that WHO's recent efforts to assist least developed countries in mobilizing external resources for health development should be expanded and lead to similar efforts by other international agencies. Thus, the focusing of attention on populations in greatest need will be increasingly applied at the international level, in addition to being a sound principle within countries.

Challenge for the future

This evaluation offers an opportunity to review and update the challenges presented at the conclusion of the second report on monitoring progress of HFA (1988). At that time five critical challenges were identified as lying in the path of progress toward health for all:

(i) **to sustain commitment** to resolve social inequities, resolve operational difficulties and expand people's responsibilities for their own health;

(ii) to intensify efforts **to expand managerial capacities**, including sound policy decision-making and focusing on priorities and targets based on valid information;

(iii) to intensify efforts **to strengthen health infrastructure** based on the principles of primary health care;

(iv) **to manage all available health resources well** while mobilizing additional resources;

(v) **to provide support to the least developed countries** on an unprecedented scale.

While this evaluation confirms that these challenges continue to be relevant, it is necessary to identify specific actions to accelerate the implementation of national and international health-for-all strategies. All such accelerating actions must address the need to improve equity in health, quality in health care, and sustainability in the national approaches employed.

They must all confirm the central role of people in health development.

(1) Sustaining commitment

The present challenge in sustaining commitment is for governments to act decisively to reduce inequity in health in specific ways. Efforts must be made to identify those populations who continue to have least access to health care and who, in all likelihood, have the greatest health needs. These population groups include the rural and urban poor, unemployed, women, children and the elderly, who may not have benefited so far from the expansion of health infrastructure. The government must also take action in areas where action by the private sector is not available. It is important to emphasize sustained commitment of people to assume greater responsibility for their health and commitment of health professionals to the principles of primary health care. The focus also needs to be sharpened to address specific health problems which mostly affect these population groups: communicable diseases such as diarrhoea, acute respiratory infection, malaria, tuberculosis and AIDS; malnutrition; and behavioural and environmental factors affecting health. Governments must establish the means to confirm their accountability to their people.

(2) Reorientation of health systems

Health care systems are in need of reorientation in specific ways. Ministries of health must closely review the breadth and focus of their responsibility and – given the concern for equity, the moves towards democratization, the realities of public sector financing and the obvious limits to the management capacity in government administrations – redefine the scope and roles of their governments in providing health care. Such redefinition must give further emphasis to disease prevention and health promotion, and focus on achieving and maintaining acceptable quality in both public and private health care and on strengthening the performance of district-level services. This reorientation must also make it easier for the community to assume more responsibility for its own health protection, in a practical, sustainable fashion. Finally, the reorientation must focus the development and management of health technology on closing the equity gap, i.e., must direct health technology development towards the health needs of vulnerable populations. Further development of human resources for health should also support this reorientation.

(3) Financing of health care

Sustaining a steady growth of resources for health implies that progress must be made in devising efficient and equitable health financing mechanisms. Funds must be assured for the operation of government programmes and services, as well as for payment by families for health care received from private sources. The trend towards an increasing role of the private health care sector will challenge all governments to implement financing schemes that address the needs of those who are least well off economically. Establishing a proper balance in health care responsibility between the government and the private sector in this manner should help to realize the redefined health role of the governments as suggested above. Financing of health care must be implemented based on considerations of equity, ethics, human rights and efficiency. In general, the resources for health must be brought closer to the people.

(4) Enhancing managerial capability

The management challenges facing government health sectors are changing. Earlier the task was to provide political advocacy for health for all, within and across sectors. Now the task is to reorient public health management to emphasize implementation. The intersectoral and intrasectoral coordinating mechanisms used for promotion, policy formulation and planning of health for all may be inappropriate for achieving broad-based action. The health sector may find it easier to play a supporting role in the programmes of other sectors, such as education, food and nutrition, and the environment. Decentralizing intersectoral action to provincial and district levels will require new styles of organization and management. The empowerment of communities to assume expanding responsibility for their own health will also entail efforts to increase their health management capabilities so that they can control better the services available to them. Management at both the decision-making and programme levels must emphasize efficiency in administration, accountability to the people, quality and improved performance in service, and should focus on priority problems and vulnerable population groups. The efforts to raise individual capacity and strengthen administrative and support systems must rely less on training and more on direct involvement in procedural improvement and problem-solving. A health information system more comprehensive in scope is needed to support such public health management.

(5) Strengthening international cooperation

While the generation of more international resources for health development will be a continuing challenge for governments and WHO, several other challenges relating to international collaboration need to be taken up. Governments and WHO must work together to improve the technical content, effectiveness, and administrative efficiency of WHO's collaboration at all levels, but particularly at the country level. Styles of collaboration must change to become more relevant, manageable and sustainable by the governments. WHO's role as the directing and coordinating authority in international

health work must be confirmed through the delivery of effective collaboration in these new styles. WHO must continue to focus attention on mobilizing resources for the least developed countries in collaboration with other agencies. In response to this new challenge in international cooperation, WHO must redefine its function and structure with a view to ensuring the rapid and realistic implementation of public health action and sustainable development.

Conclusion

This evaluation has relied on: extensive work done in countries to compile data and assess progress; efforts at the WHO regional offices to summarize the country submissions and make intercountry comparisons; and the analysis at the global level which produced the overall summary of major trends and constraints. In addition to providing this benchmark on the road to health for all, it is hoped this global evaluation effort will contribute substantially to the definition of a new framework for public health action. Such a framework must facilitate sustainable health development directed towards:

- developing and appropriately distributing the resources (financial, human and technological) that are required for addressing priority health needs;
- achieving equity in health status by undertaking more effective health promotion and protection, most of which takes place in sectors other than health; and
- pursuing equality in access to primary health care employing increasingly integrated and high-quality services.

This second evaluation of the global strategy, which focuses health development clearly on people, has consequences for health policy in all countries and implications for the work of international agencies, particularly WHO, in order to achieve **effective implementation** of the health-for-all strategies.

Statistical annex

1. Global indicators for monitoring and evaluating progress

In order to monitor and evaluate progress in the implementation of health-for-all strategies, WHO's Member States have agreed to provide information periodically on a set of global indicators devised for this purpose. These indicators were reviewed in 1990 by the Executive Board, which approved a revised list of indicators and new definitions, particularly for the second strategy evaluation in 1991. The list includes three **new** indicators: the percentage of women of child-bearing age using family planning, maternal mortality rate and the probability of dying before the age of 5 years (i.e., under-5 mortality) introduced for the first time for the second evaluation. Some of the indicators, such as adequate excreta-disposal facilities, were reformulated and a few were redefined (e.g., antenatal coverage). The changes are listed below.

List of reformulated global indicators

The proposed reformulations, arrived at by consensus between technical programmes at headquarters and the regions and adopted with amendments by the Executive Board by resolution EB85.R5, are shown below. Changes from the original versions are in bold print.

No. 1　The number of countries in which health for all **is continuing to** receive endorsement as policy at the highest level.

No. 2　The number of countries in which mechanisms for involving people in the implementation of strategies **are fully functioning or are being further developed**.

No. 3　**The percentage** of gross national product spent on health.

No. 4　**The** percentage of the national health expenditure devoted to local health **services**.

No. 5　The number of countries in which re-

sources for primary health care **are becoming more** equitably distributed.

No. 6　**The amount of international aid received or given for health.**

No. 7　**The percentage of** the population **covered** by primary health care, with at least the following:

– safe water in the home or **with reasonable access**, and adequate **excreta-disposal** facilities **available**;

– immunization against diphtheria, tetanus, whooping-cough, measles, poliomyelitis, and tuberculosis;

– local health **services**, including availability of essential drugs, within one hour's walk or travel;

– **attendance by** trained personnel for pregnancy and childbirth, and caring for children up to at least 1 year of age.

The percentage of women of child-bearing age using family planning.

The percentage of each element should be given for all identifiable subgroups.

No. 8　**The percentage of newborns weighing** at least 2500 grams **at birth**, and **the percentage of children whose** weight-for-age **and/or weight-for-height are acceptable**.

No. 9　The infant mortality rate (IMR), **maternal mortality rate (MMR) and probability of dying before the age of 5 years ($q5$)**, in all identifiable subgroups.

No. 10　Life expectancy at birth, **by sex, in all identifiable subgroups**.

No. 11　The adult literacy rate, **by sex, in all identifiable subgroups**.

No. 12　The **per capita** gross national product.

These indicators were incorporated in a *Common framework for the second evaluation* (CFE/2), prepared to assist Member States in carrying out the evaluation of implementation of their national strategies. Even though the indicators are considered to be the minimum necessary to assess progress with overall health development, the statistical infrastructure required to obtain the data is not yet operative in many countries, reflecting the logistic and financial difficulties associated with the installation of an adequate health information system. In order to provide maximum information support to health-for-all strategy implementation, the data collected must be representative, accurate, and timely.

2. Explanatory notes

Of the 168 Member States, 151 communicated their findings to WHO and provided data/information on some or all of these global indicators. It should be noted that information on the percentage of the population covered by all elements of primary health care (global indicator 7) is not available. This indicator comprises four selected elements of PHC, each of which may comprise several subelements (e.g., the fourth element of the indicator actually comprises two subelements: attendance by trained personnel for pregnancy and childbirth, and caring for children up to at least 1 year of age). Data are not always available for all the subelements, but only for one aspect of one subelement (e.g., trained personnel for childbirth). Similarly, data may be available for safe water and excreta-disposal facilities separately, but not necessarily for both subelements. Thus in a number of cases, data were provided for some sub-indicators or subelements only and not for the relevant global indicator.

For the first time in connection with the monitoring and evaluation of health-for-all strategies, the global review (based primarily on the national and regional reports) has analysed the availability and timeliness of data on the global indicators reported by Member States. Data on global indicators are available in the respective regional reports/syntheses and hence are not given here.

It has been noted that the majority of Member States are still experiencing great difficulty in obtaining valid and timely data on key health indicators. As a result, it is extremely difficult to derive overall estimates of indicator values in order to assess progress at the global level. For this purpose, it has been necessary to prepare estimates of the indicator values for major groups of countries and the world as a whole by drawing on information from other sources. These include the data collected and reviewed by WHO technical programmes, other international agencies such as UNESCO, the World Bank, the United Nations (in particular the Population Division), as well as on the research reports and data bases of other institutions. On this basis, estimates have been prepared for the two periods 1983–1985 and 1988–1990, corresponding to the periods covered respectively by the first evaluation of the strategies for HFA in 1985 and the second in 1991.

The estimates of infant mortality and life expectancy are based on estimates prepared by the United Nations in 1990 for 146 of the 168 WHO Member States with populations greater than 300 000 in 1990. Demographic indicators for populations below this size tend to be affected by large annual variations in births and deaths and hence no estimates were available. The smaller Member States of WHO together account for about 2 650 000 people or about 0.05% of the world`s population.

For analytical purposes, the following country classifications as proposed by the United Nations have been used for grouping the Member States. It should be noted however that the designations used in this publication are those which were applicable during the period 1985–1990, which is covered by this evaluation.

Developing countries:

Latin America and the Caribbean, Africa (excluding South Africa), Asia and the Pacific (excluding Australia, Japan and New Zealand), Cyprus, Malta and Yugoslavia.

of which *least developed countries (as of June 1991)*

> Afghanistan, Bangladesh, Benin, Bhutan, Botswana, Burkina Faso, Burundi, Cape Verde, Central African Republic, Chad, Comoros, Djibouti, Equatorial Guinea, Ethiopia, Gambia, Guinea, Guinea-Bissau, Haiti, Kiribati, Lao People's Democratic Republic, Lesotho, Liberia, Malawi, Maldives, Mali, Mauritania, Mozambique, Myanmar, Nepal, Niger, Rwanda, Samoa, Sao Tome and Principe, Sierra Leone, Somalia, Sudan, Togo, Uganda, United Republic of Tanzania, Vanuatu and Yemen.

Eastern Europe:

> Albania, Bulgaria, Byelorussian SSR, Czechoslovakia, Hungary, Poland, Romania, Ukrainian SSR and the USSR.

Developed market

> North America, northern, southern and western Europe (excluding Cyprus, Malta and Yugoslavia), Australia, Japan, New Zealand and South Africa.

The above designations of country groups in the text and the tables are intended solely for statistical and analytical convenience and do not necessarily express a judgement about the stage reached by a particular country in the development process.

The reported and estimated values of (or information on) each HFA global indicator according to broad development groups for the first evaluation in 1985 and the second in 1991 are given in the Annex table. In the tables, values under **1985** refer to the period 1983–1985 and under **1991** to 1988–1990. Data are presented for each of the three main country groupings – developing countries (with one sub-grouping – least developed countries), eastern European countries and developed market economies, as well as for the world as a whole. Data for Yemen and former Democratic Yemen as well as for the former German Democratic

Republic and the Federal Republic of Germany are included separately for the computations of the weighted values, since the data refer to the period prior to the merger and unification. However, the respective populations of these countries have been added together accordingly to reflect these changes in the tables. The estimates or reported data for each of the country groupings are weighted values of the estimates or reported data for each country in that group, with the weighting procedure given in a footnote to the table. Furthermore, for each of the two periods, the number of Member States in each country grouping reporting data or information, together with the respective percentage of the population included in computing the weighted averages, is shown along with the reported or estimated indicator value. Not all data provided for the second evaluation could be used to compute the weighted values for 1991, because some of them applied to years previous to the period 1988–1990. For comparative purposes, the weighted values for 1985 shown in the Annex table were based on data covering the period 1983–1985 only. For some indicators, such as infant mortality, the weighted averages are based on almost 100% coverage of Member States owing to the availability of national estimates from other sources. In other cases, for example the care of pregnant women by trained personnel, there is no consolidated set of national estimates other than the data reported by Member States in their evaluation reports, and so the coverage of countries for that indicator is considerably less than 100%.

Even though efforts have been made to arrive at a set of comparable values for different global indicators for assessing progress since the first evaluation in 1985, the weighted values for the four groups of countries considered can at best be considered reasonable estimates giving the direction of progress, and not precise values appropriate for rigorous analysis.

Annex table. Global indicators 1-12[a]

Global indicator 1 - HFA endorsement continues

Country groupings	Number of Member States	1991 population (millions)	Number of Member States responding positively[1] 1991	Population included, 1991[2] (%)
Developing countries	132	4 142	96	91
of which:				
least developed	*41*	*460*	*33*	*90*
Eastern Europe	9	391	2	12
Developed market economies	27	837	12	51
Total	168	5 370	110	79

[1] Out of 168 Member States, 151 reported, of which: 110 provided a positive response; 4 provided a negative response; 37 did not provide the required information, or any information.
[2] Population included: 4 230 million or 79% of the total population of all Member States.

Global indicator 2 - Community involvement: mechanisms fully functioning / being further developed

Country groupings	Number of Member States	1991 population (millions)	Number of Member States responding positively[1] 1991	Population included, 1991[2] (%)
Developing countries	132	4 142	82	84
of which:				
least developed	*41*	*460*	*29*	*52*
Eastern Europe	9	391	1	10
Developed market economies	27	837	11	51
Total	168	5 370	94	73

[1] Out of 168 Member States, 151 reported, of which: 94 provided a positive response; 7 provided a negative response; 50 did not provide the required information, or any information.
[2] Population included: 3 936 million or 73% of the total population of all Member States.

Global indicator 3 - Percentage of GNP spent on health
(Central government expenditure on health as percentage of GNP)

Country groupings	Number of Member States	1991 population (millions)	Weighted value (%) 1991[1]	1985	Number of Member States included, 1991	Population included 1991[2] (%)	Number of Member States included, 1985	Population included 1985[3] (%)
Developing countries	132	4 142	0.9	0.9	42	42	69	59
of which:								
least developed	*41*	*460*	*1.4*	*1.0*	*5*	*9*	*16*	*61*
Eastern Europe	9	391	1.2	2.0	1	3	1	3
Developed market economies	27	837	3.3	3.8	14	57	22	80
Total	168	5 370	3.0	3.3	57	41	92	58

[1] Based on values for 57 Member States and weighted by their respective gross national product.
[2] Population included: 2 218 million or 41% of the total population of all Member States.
[3] Population included: 2 801 million or 58% of the total population of all Member States.

[a] Information reported by Member States for the 1985 and 1991 evaluations are used for global indicators 1, 2, 4, 5, 6, 7.5, 7.6, 7.7, 7.8, 7.9 and 8; WHO estimates are used for global indicators 3, 7.1, 7.2, 7.3, 7.4, 9, 10, 11 and 12. Only those Member States for which data are available for the period 1988-1990 are included for computation related to the 1991 evaluation, and only those for which data are available for the period 1983-1985 are included for the 1985 evaluation.

Global indicator 4 - Percentage of national health expenditure devoted to local health services

Country groupings	Number of Member States	1991 population (millions)	Weighted value (%) 1991[1]	1985	Number of Member States reporting, 1991[2]	Population included 1991[3] (%)	Number of Member States included, 1985	Population included 1985[4] (%)
Developing countries	132	4 142	28	32	47	36	61	77
of which:								
least developed	*41*	*460*	*37*	*39*	*16*	*25*	*27*	*73*
Eastern Europe	9	391	...	40	0	..	3	9
Developed market economies	27	837	16	25	3	11	10	27
Total	168	5 370	18	25	50	29	74	63

[1] Based on values for 50 Member States and weighted by their respective health expenditures.
[2] Out of 168 Member States, 151 reported, of which: 50 provided data referring to the period 1988-90; 26 provided data referring to other periods; 75 did not provide the required information, or any information.
[3] Population included: 1 579 million or 29% of the total population of all Member States.
[4] Population included: 3 067 million or 63% of the total population of all Member States.

Global indicator 5 - Resources for primary health care: equitable distribution

Country groupings	Number of Member States	1991 population (millions)	Number of Member States responding positively[1] 1991	Population included, 1991[2] (%)
Developing countries	132	4 142	27	44
of which:				
least developed	*41*	*460*	*7*	*24*
Eastern Europe	9	391	1	3
Developed market economies	27	837	4	3
Total	168	5 370	32	34

[1] Out of 168 Member States, 151 reported, of which: 32 provided a positive response; 11 provided a negative response; 108 did not provide the required information, or any information.
[2] Population included: 1 851 million or 34% of the total population of all Member States.

Global indicator 6.1 - Aid received for health (US$)

Data available from OECD member countries only.

Global indicator 6.2 - Aid given for health (US$)

Data available for OECD member countries only.

Global indicator 7.1 - Safe water: population coverage

Country groupings	Number of Member States	1991 population (millions)	Weighted value (%) 1991[1]	1985	Number of Member States included, 1991	Population included 1991[2] (%)	Number of Member States included, 1985	Population included 1985[3] (%)
Developing countries	132	4 142	68	55	86	64	85	61
of which:								
least developed	*41*	*460*	*49*	*30*	*29*	*83*	*26*	*62*
Eastern Europe	9	391	100	98	8	100	6	93
Developed-market economies	27	837	100	100	22	45	14	66
Total	168	5 370	75	68	116	64	105	65

[1] Based on values for 116 Member States and weighted by their respective total population.
[2] Population included: 3 445 million or 64% of the total population of all Member States.
[3] Population included: 3 137 million or 65% of the total population of all Member States.

Global indicator 7.2 - Adequate excreta-disposal facilities: population coverage

Country groupings	Number of Member States	1991 population (millions)	Weighted value (%)		Number of Member States included, 1991	Population included 1991[2] (%)	Number of Member States included, 1985	Population included 1985[3] (%)
			1991[1]	1985				
Developing countries	132	4 142	56	31	68	29	75	61
of which:								
least developed	*41*	*460*	*23*	*14*	*20*	*71*	*24*	*81*
Eastern Europe	9	391	100	100	5	93	6	93
Developed market economies	27	837	100	100	18	35	11	32
Total	168	5 370	71	46	91	35	92	59

[1] Based on values for 91 Member States and weighted by their respective total population.
[2] Population included: 1 870 million or 35% of the total population of all Member States.
[3] Population included: 2 858 million or 59% of the total population of all Member States.

Global indicator 7.3.1 - Six EPI diseases: percentage of infants immunized

Data not available.

Global indicator 7.3.2 - Immunization of infants: coverage by DPT vaccine

Country groupings	Number of Member States	1991 population (millions)	Weighted value (%)		Number of Member States included, 1991	Population included 1991[2] (%)	Number of Member States included, 1985	Population included 1985[3] (%)
			1991[1]	1985				
Developing countries	132	4 142	83	41	131	100	121	98
of which:								
least developed	*41*	*460*	*69*	*16*	*41*	*100*	*35*	*91*
Eastern Europe	9	391	75	90	8	100	8	100
Developed market economies	27	837	88	79	27	100	23	92
Total	168	5 370	83	47	166	100	152	97

[1] Based on values for 166 Member States and weighted by their respective number of live births.
[2] Population included: 5 368 million or 100% of the total population of all Member States.
[3] Population included: 4 710 million or 97% of the total population of all Member States.

Global indicator 7.3.3 - Immunization of infants: coverage by measles vaccine

Country groupings	Number of Member States	1991 population (millions)	Weighted value (%)		Number of Member States included, 1991	Population included 1991[2] (%)	Number of Member States included, 1985	Population included 1985[3] (%)
			1991[1]	1985				
Developing countries	132	4 142	79	44	131	100	114	75
of which:								
least developed	*41*	*460*	*43*	*26*	*41*	*100*	*33*	*82*
Eastern Europe	9	391	87	86	8	100	6	87
Developed market economies	27	837	80	72	26	100	19	89
Total	168	5 370	80	50	165	100	139	78

[1] Based on values for 165 Member States and weighted by their respective number of live births.
[2] Population included: 5 368 million or 100% of the total population of all Member States.
[3] Population included: 3 771 million or 78% of the total population of all Member States.

Global indicator 7.3.4 - Immunization of infants: coverage by poliomyelitis vaccine

Country groupings	Number of Member States	1991 population (millions)	Weighted value (%)		Number of Member States included, 1991	Population included 1991[2] (%)	Number of Member States included, 1985	Population included 1985[3] (%)
			1991[1]	1985				
Developing countries	132	4 142	85	43	131	100	116	97
of which:								
least developed	41	460	62	14	41	100	33	89
Eastern Europe	9	391	80	94	8	100	8	100
Developed market economies	27	837	90	91	27	100	23	92
Total	168	5 370	85	50	166	100	147	97

[1] Based on values for 166 Member States and weighted by their respective number of live births.
[2] Population included: 5 368 million or 100% of the total population of all Member States.
[3] Population included: 4 682 million or 97% of the total population of all Member States.

Global indicator 7.3.5 - Immunization of infants: coverage by BCG vaccine

Country groupings	Number of Member States	1991 population (millions)	Weighted value (%)		Number of Member States included, 1991	Population included 1991[2] (%)	Number of Member States included, 1985	Population included 1985[3] (%)
			1991[1]	1985				
Developing countries	132	4 142	90	42	117	98	108	98
of which:								
least developed	41	460	79	27	41	100	34	91
Eastern Europe	9	391	93	93	7	94	7	94
Developed market economies	27	837	80	65	13	46	15	51
Total	168	5 370	90	45	137	90	130	90

[1] Based on values for 137 Member States and weighted by their respective number of live births.
[2] Population included: 4 828 million or 90% of the total population of all Member States.
[3] Population included: 4 346 million or 90% of the total population of all Member States.

Global indicator 7.4 - Immunization of pregnant women: coverage by tetanus toxoid vaccine

Country groupings	Number of Member States	1991 population (millions)	Weighted value (%)		Number of Member States included, 1991	Population included 1991[2] (%)	Number of Member States included, 1985	Population included 1985[3] (%)
			1991[1]	1985				
Developing countries	132	4 142	39	24	103	67	74	81
of which:								
least developed	41	460	37	10	40	99	32	89
Eastern Europe	9	391	...	...	0	..	0	..
Developed market economies	27	837	...	...	0	..	0	..
Total	168	5 370	34	24	103	52	74	61

[1] Based on values for 103 Member States and weighted by their respective number of live births.
[2] Population included: 2 767 million or 52% of the total population of all Member States.
[3] Population included: 2 962 million or 61% of the total population of all Member States.

Global indicator 7.5 - Local health services: population coverage

Country groupings	Number of Member States	1991 population (millions)	Weighted value (%) 1991[1]	1985	Number of Member States reporting, 1991[2]	Population included 1991[3] (%)	Number of Member States included, 1985	Population included 1985[4] (%)
Developing countries	132	4 142	89	70	33	38	75	43
of which:								
least developed	*41*	*460*	*69*	*48*	*11*	*52*	*29*	*87*
Eastern Europe	9	391	...	100	0	..	9	91
Developed market economies	27	837	100	100	3	16	18	81
Total	168	5 370	90	81	36	32	102	53

[1] Based on values for 36 Member States and weighted by their respective total population.
[2] Out of 168 Member States, 151 reported, of which: 36 provided data referring to the period 1988-90; 34 provided data referring to other periods; 81 did not provide the required information, or any information.
[3] Population included: 1 702 million or 32% of the total population of all Member States.
[4] Population included: 2 553 million or 53% of the total population of all Member States.

Global indicator 7.6 - Prenatal care: coverage by trained personnel

Country groupings	Number of Member States	1991 population (millions)	Weighted value (per 100 live births) 1991[1]	1985	Number of Member States reporting, 1991[2]	Population included 1991[3] (%)	Number of Member States included, 1985	Population included 1985[4] (%)
Developing countries	132	4 142	65	48	61	46	67	43
of which:								
least developed	*41*	*460*	*53*	*45*	*22*	*65*	*22*	*51*
Eastern Europe	9	391	...	100	0	..	6	83
Developed market economies	27	837	99	96	3	46	12	61
Total	168	5 370	67	58	64	42	85	49

[1] Based on values for 64 Member States and weighted by their respective number of live births.
[2] Out of 168 Member States, 151 reported, of which: 64 provided data referring to the period 1988-90; 27 provided data referring to other periods; 60 did not provide the required information, or any information.
[3] Population included: 2 280 million or 42% of the total population of all Member States.
[4] Population included: 2 387 million or 49% of the total population of all Member States.

Global indicator 7.7 - Childbirth attendance: coverage by trained personnel

Country groupings	Number of Member States	1991 population (millions)	Weighted value (per 100 live births) 1991[1]	1985	Number of Member States reporting, 1991[2]	Population included 1991[3] (%)	Number of Member States included, 1985	Population included 1985[4] (%)
Developing countries	132	4 142	53	41	63	79	76	46
of which:								
least developed	*41*	*460*	*32*	*36*	*19*	*57*	*22*	*56*
Eastern Europe	9	391	...	100	0	..	7	84
Developed market economies	27	837	99	99	5	47	14	72
Total	168	5 370	55	53	68	68	97	53

[1] Based on values for 68 Member States and weighted by their respective number of live births.
[2] Out of 168 Member States, 151 reported, of which: 68 provided data referring to the period 1988-90; 26 provided data referring to other periods; 57 did not provide the required information, or any information.
[3] Population included: 3 654 million or 68% of the total population of all Member States.
[4] Population included: 2 562 million or 53% of the total population of all Member States.

Global indicator 7.8 - Infant care: coverage by trained personnel

Country groupings	Number of Member States	1991 population (millions)	Weighted value (per 100 live births) 1991[1]	1985	Number of Member States reporting, 1991[2]	Population included 1991[3] (%)	Number of Member States included, 1985	Population included 1985[4] (%)
Developing countries	132	4 142	64	43	47	48	53	15
of which:								
least developed	41	460	56	36	13	43	13	41
Eastern Europe	9	391	...	99	0	..	7	84
Developed market economies	27	837	100	98	1	0	11	25
Total	168	5 370	64	60	48	37	71	22

[1] Based on values for 48 Member States and weighted by their respective number of live births.
[2] Out of 168 Member States, 151 reported, of which: 48 provided data referring to the period 1988-90; 21 provided data referring to other periods; 82 did not provide the required information, or any information.
[3] Population included: 1 977 million or 37% of the total population of all Member States.
[4] Population included: 1 084 million or 22% of the total population of all Member States.

Global indicator 7.9 - Contraceptive use: coverage of women of child-bearing age

Country groupings	Number of Member States	1991 population (millions)	Weighted value 1991[1] (%)	Number of Member States reporting, 1991[2]	Population included, 1991[3] (%)
Developing countries	132	4 142	34	53	41
of which:					
least developed	41	460	8	20	22
Eastern Europe	9	391	...	0	..
Developed market economies	27	837	61	2	37
Total	168	5 370	38	55	37

[1] Based on values for 55 Member States and weighted by their respective female population aged 15-49 years.
[2] Out of 168 Member States, 151 reported, of which: 55 provided data referring to the period 1988-90; 26 provided data referring to other periods; 70 did not provide the required information, or any information.
[3] Population included: 2 000 million or 37% of the total population of all Member States.

Global indicator 8.1 - Birthweight: percentage of newborns weighing at least 2500 grams

Country groupings	Number of Member States	1991 population (millions)	Weighted value (%) 1991[1]	1985	Number of Member States reporting, 1991[2]	Population included 1991[3] (%)	Number of Member States included, 1985	Population included 1985[4] (%)
Developing countries	132	4 142	87	78	55	53	64	44
of which:								
least developed	41	460	76	88	19	52	19	42
Eastern Europe	9	391	94	93	4	87	6	20
Developed market economies	27	837	93	94	13	55	15	39
Total	168	5 370	88	79	72	56	85	41

[1] Based on values for 72 Member States and weighted by their respective number of live births.
[2] Out of 168 Member States, 151 reported, of which: 72 provided data referring to the period 1988-90; 38 provided data referring to other periods; 41 did not provide the required information, or any information.
[3] Population included: 2 996 million or 56% of the total population of all Member States.
[4] Population included: 2 005 million or 41% of the total population of all Member States.

Global indicator 8.2 - Acceptable weight for age: percentage of children

Data not available.

Global indicator 9.1 - Infant mortality rate

Country groupings	Number of Member States	1991 population (millions)	Weighted value (per 1000 live births) 1991[1]	1985	Number of Member States included, 1991	Population included 1991[2] (%)	Number of Member States included, 1985	Population included 1985[3] (%)
Developing countries	132	4 142	75	86	113	100	113	100
of which:								
least developed	*41*	*460*	*119*	*130*	*37*	*100*	*37*	*100*
Eastern Europe	9	391	22	24	8	100	8	100
Developed market economies	27	837	14	16	25	100	25	100
Total	168	5 370	68	76	146	100	146	100

[1] Based on values for 146 Member States and weighted by their respective number of live births.
[2] Population included: 5 368 million or 100% of the total population of all Member States.
[3] Population included: 4 836 million or 100% of the total population of all Member States.

Global indicator 9.2 - Maternal mortality rate

Country groupings	Number of Member States	1991 population (millions)	Weighted value 1991[1] (per 100 000 live births)	Number of Member States included, 1991	Population included, 1991[2] (%)
Developing countries	132	4 142	421	113	100
of which:					
least developed	*41*	*460*	*737*	*37*	*100*
Eastern Europe	9	391	41	8	100
Developed market economies	27	837	34	25	100
Total	168	5 370	370	146	100

[1] Based on values for 146 Member States and weighted by their respective number of live births.
[2] Population included: 5 368 million or 100% of the total population of all Member States.

Global indicator 9.3 - Under-five mortality rate (probability of dying before age five)

Country groupings	Number of Member States	1991 population (millions)	Weighted value 1991[1] (per 1000 live births)	Number of Member States included	Population included, 1991[2] (%)
Developing countries	132	4 142	117	112	100
of which:					
least developed	*41*	*460*	*198*	*36*	*100*
Eastern Europe	9	391	25	8	100
Developed market economies	27	837	18	25	100
Total	168	5 370	104	145	100

[1] Based on values for 145 Member States and weighted by their respective number of live births.
[2] Population included: 5 368 million or 100% of the total population of all Member States.

Global indicator 10 - Life expectancy at birth (both sexes)

Country groupings	Number of Member States	1991 population (millions)	Weighted value (years) 1991[1]	1985	Number of Member States included, 1991	Population included 1991[2] (%)	Number of Member States included, 1985	Population included 1985[3] (%)
Developing countries *of which:*	132	4 142	62	61	113	100	113	100
least developed	41	460	50	48	37	100	37	100
Eastern Europe	9	391	71	69	8	100	8	100
Developed market economies	27	837	76	75	25	100	25	100
Total	168	5 370	65	64	146	100	146	100

[1] Based on values for 146 Member States and weighted by their respective total population.
[2] Population included: 5 368 million or 100% of the total population of all Member States.
[3] Population included: 4 836 million or 100% of the total population of all Member States.

Global indicator 11 - Adult literacy rate

Country groupings	Number of Member States	1991 population (millions)	Weighted value (%) 1991[1]	1985	Number of Member States included, 1991	Population included 1991[2] (%)	Number of Member States included, 1985	Population included 1985[3] (%)
Developing countries *of which:*	132	4 142	65	61	90	97	90	97
least developed	41	460	40	36	29	79	29	79
Eastern Europe	9	391	...	...	0	..	0	..
Developed market economies	27	837	95	94	4	14	4	15
Total	168	5 370	66	62	94	77	94	75

[1] Based on values for 94 Member States and weighted by their respective population aged 15 years and above.
[2] Population included: 4 119 million or 77% of the total population of all Member States.
[3] Population included: 3 649 million or 75% of the total population of all Member States.

Global indicator 12 - Per capita gross national product (US$)

Country groupings	Number of Member States	1991 population (millions)	Weighted value (US$) 1991[1]	1985	Number of Member States included, 1991	Population included 1991[2] (%)	Number of Member States included, 1985	Population included 1985[3] (%)
Developing countries *of which:*	132	4 142	700	659	105	91	106	93
least developed	41	460	219	197	32	81	32	82
Eastern Europe	9	391	1 931	2 049	2	12	2	12
Developed market economies	27	837	17 777	11 423	25	100	25	100
Total	168	5 370	3 727	2 692	132	87	133	88

[1] Based on values for 132 Member States and weighted by their respective total population.
[2] Population included: 4 653 million or 87% of the total population of all Member States.
[3] Population included: 4 236 million or 88% of the total population of all Member States.

Index

Main references are in bold type